FAT COW, FAT CHANCE

FAT Cow, FAT Chance

THE SCIENCE AND PSYCHOLOGY OF SIZE

JENNI MURRAY

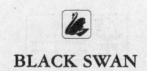

BLACK SWAN

TRANSWORLD PUBLISHERS
Penguin Random House, One Embassy Gardens,
8 Viaduct Gardens, London SW11 7BW
www.penguin.co.uk

Transworld is part of the Penguin Random House group of companies
whose addresses can be found at global.penguinrandomhouse.com

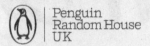

Penguin
Random House
UK

First published in Great Britain in 2020 by Doubleday
an imprint of Transworld Publishers
Black Swan edition published 2021

A CIP catalogue record for this book
is available from the British Library.

ISBN
9781784163969

Typeset in 10.81/14.08pt Minion Pro by Jouve (UK), Milton Keynes.
Printed and bound in Great Britain by Clays Ltd, Elcograf S.p.A.

The authorized representative in the EEA is Penguin Random House Ireland,
Morrison Chambers, 32 Nassau Street, Dublin D02 YH68.

Penguin Random House is committed to a sustainable
future for our business, our readers and our planet. This book
is made from Forest Stewardship Council® certified paper.

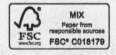

This book is dedicated to Professor Francesco Rubino,
who changed my life.

Contents

Introduction

I can't begin to tell you how many times I've been walking down the street, minding my own business, pottering along on my bike or simply sitting in a queue of traffic at the wheel of my Mini when, apropos of absolutely nothing, I've heard 'fat cow', 'fat bitch', sometimes 'fat c***' (sorry, can't bring myself to actually write that one) or, 'Eh, love, who ate all the pies?'

Every time it happened I would try to convince myself I didn't care.

Yes, for much of my adult life I was substantially overweight, obese even, and had done every diet known to man or woman with no lasting success. I'd done my very best to persuade myself that it was possible to be fat and happy, and that the people who loved me wouldn't cease to care just because the middle-age spread had got somewhat out of control.

By the time I was sixty-four years old my weight had become quite crippling. I told myself my obesity had played no role in the breast cancer I'd been diagnosed with in 2006 (almost certainly wrong) and that my need for a bilateral hip replacement had nothing to do with the strain I'd been putting on my joints. I put all the blame for the damage done to my bones on the chemotherapy I had after the cancer surgery.

For so long I had wanted to join the ever-increasing groups of women – Dawn French, Jo Brand, Beth Ditto, Rebel Wilson and, most recently, Sofie Hagen, the author of *Happy Fat* – who argued it was possible to be fat and fit, and were furious at the fat shaming that is so widespread. Hagen claims to have become completely at ease with 'taking up space in a world that wants to shrink you'.

The excuses I made to myself were legion. I was, I kept on telling myself, fat and happy and I didn't care about the insults. The fat part was blatantly obvious. The happy was an Oscar-winning performance put on in public, but in private I lived with a growing sense of fear and misery that this incredible hulk was my lot for evermore and would probably kill me long before I reached my three score years and ten. I did care, but for so long I tried to put all the worries to the back of my mind.

I tended to avoid the scales and merrily ordered clothes online from the Sixteen47 website owned by Dawn French and Helen Teague, which boasts 'the biggest range of plus sizes in the UK'. I wore only their baggiest tops in the most voluminous size along with a pair of stretchy leggings – always a 'slimming' black in colour. I joked I'd managed to create a uniform for myself that made life so much easier in the morning.

It was just like school days, I told myself. I didn't have to think about what I was going to wear. My mind could be occupied with more important thoughts than the frivolity of fashion. I simply needed to make sure there were plenty of the same type of items in the wardrobe so all I had to do was pick out a clean outfit. Ordering online meant never having to go into a shop and face the disapproving glances of a sales assistant who doubted she would have anything in my size, and never having to endure the humiliation of a communal changing room.

So, I simply used the uniform to hide away all the abundant flesh and, at the same time, tried hard to become immune to what I was feeling about the constant insults. Some days I would let the anger bubble to the surface and shout back some foul obscenity. Witty remarks never seemed to come to me at those horrible moments. Mostly, I wanted only to curl up and die. Go home and eat something comforting. And that, of course, was no solution to the problem.

Two things shocked me into taking myself in hand. My old GP, who was also significantly overweight, retired. I guess I'd always used her as an excuse. If my doctor was fat, what did I have to worry about? She never made me step on the scales and I don't recall her ever suggesting weight loss might be a good idea. I should, perhaps, point out that, like me, she also had breast cancer – in her case twice.

My new GP is a man. He's quite elderly and never pulls his punches. He suggested I step on the scales at our first appointment. The scales groaned and so did I when I saw the reason why. Twenty-four stone! How on earth had I allowed that to happen? My doctor's question was what did I propose to do about it?

The second shock came when my son Charlie accompanied me and my three little dogs on a walk in the local park. My walks tended to be slow, painful and rather lumbering, with frequent pauses at benches. We were having a 'little sit-down' when an enormous woman passed us, driving a mobility scooter. Her two dogs trotted along beside her, their leads attached to the handlebar. 'Blimey, Mum,' said Charlie, his voice full of concern, 'if you aren't careful, that'll be you before long.'

It was the prompt I needed to do something about it. This book tells the story of how I took that fat chance, lost 8 stone in less than a year and how my weight has now stabilized as I've developed a healthy relationship with food without losing the pleasure I take in eating it. It also asks why obesity is the health crisis it has become and explains how the food and diet industries have done us anything but good. I hope the second part of the book's title indicates a new interpretation of the expression 'fat chance' – no longer a negative, but a positive opportunity to get well again at a healthy weight.

I've kept the 'fat cow' in the first part because the stigma directed at so many of us simply has to be tackled. It was not until I attended a symposium on obesity and stigma in 2017 that one of the speakers, Dr Stuart Flint, made a point that opened my eyes to what those of us who suffer from obesity have to endure. 'Hate speech,' he said, 'is illegal and a number of conditions are covered by the law. Expressions of hatred towards someone on account of the person's colour, race, disability, nationality, ethnic or national origin, religion, gender identity or sexual orientation are illegal. Any communication which is threatening or abusive and is intended to harass, alarm or distress someone is forbidden. The penalties for hate speech include fines, imprisonment or both. However,' he paused, 'you will note there is one common condition which frequently induces what I would describe as hate speech that is not included in the list. And that condition is obesity.'

It was a profound moment for me. A light bulb began to flash in my brain, prompting me to do something to spread the word that fat shaming is hate speech, even though it's not included in the statutes. For the person who hears it, it is insulting and deeply distressing. People will often justify calling out to the 'fat cow', making the assumption that, whilst it's impossible and undesirable to change your colour, race, disability or chosen gender identity, the fat person should want to change their physical form and, indeed, could change it if they weren't so greedy and lazy.

You'll often hear the mantra 'take less energy in and put more energy out'. Most thin people who haven't suffered the struggle with a body that refuses to conform to what's thought to be the norm – slimness – assume you can successfully go on a regime of diet and exercise and no longer be an obese, sick drain on the NHS, suffering from type 2 diabetes, heart trouble and some cancers. It's worth pointing out at this stage that even thin people have diabetes, cancer and cardiac arrests, but you wouldn't think so from the daily diet of news stories describing an obesity epidemic.

Over the past year alone I have counted hundreds of headlines in various newspapers warning of the risks and general downside of becoming overweight: 'Generation fat: 40 per cent of young are overweight', 'Children who are obese at eleven "being doomed to an early death"', 'Diabetes cases double in just twenty years', 'Britons eating 50 per cent more than they say', 'Children face obesity apocalypse', 'Bad lifestyles to blame for 2,500 cancer cases per week', 'Give patients crash diets on NHS says Oxford professor', 'Blobbie Williams no more! Slimline star is now a Weight Watchers ambassador', 'Why don't chubby stars get any sex scenes?', 'Gorging into the grave', 'One new diabetes case every three minutes', 'Obesity is the new smoking', 'New war on junk food', 'Skipping breakfast is making children fat', 'Huge health risks of high BMI', 'Pill that expands in stomach doubles weight-loss chance'. OK! Enough! You get the picture.

My intention in writing this book is to explain what it feels like to be fat and how incredibly difficult it is to lose the weight, no matter how hard you try. I shall also try to unpick the complex new scientific discoveries that explain why going on a diet is rarely the answer to the fat girl or boy's problems. In recent years, science has come on apace to increase understanding of the genetic, environmental, evolutionary and metabolic reasons why some of us can eat as many chips as we choose without putting on an ounce and some of us will balloon if we dare to walk past a chippy and merely sniff, without consuming so much as one fry.

I would like to think that people who read this book and discuss its contents will begin to understand why fat shaming is so hurtful, harmful and cruel. The stigma often makes fat people withdraw into themselves to the extent they are too afraid even to go to a doctor to discuss the problem and enquire what solutions there might be.

My aim is never, ever to hear any passing stranger call out 'fat cow' to anyone. Never again.

1

The First Taste

May 1950 and my mother – a slim and really rather gorgeous twenty-four-year-old woman called Win – is taken off to hospital in her husband Alvin's best friend's Wolseley as her contractions begin. The new maternity hospital in Barnsley, St Helen's, is a former workhouse and somewhat forbidding Victorian grey-stone construction. But it's all going to be fine. The NHS is only two years old and the excited but frightened mother-to-be is full of confidence that she'll receive the very latest in modern maternity care, which won't cost her and her impecunious man a penny.

Her subsequent stories of how ghastly the whole procedure was have stayed with me throughout my life. It's an object lesson in how much of our future – our habits, beliefs and anxieties – is formulated in early childhood, and often as a result of the tales told by our parents and grandparents. My mother was shaved, given an enema and left alone with her legs up in stirrups for a labour that lasted more than twenty-four hours. As both she and I were on the point of expiry, a consultant obstetrician came on duty, popped into the delivery room, recognized impending disaster and whipped me out with forceps.

No wonder she'd had so many problems trying to give birth

to me. She'd been lying on her back for all that time with nothing but gas and air to ease her pain. She had not been blessed with the childbearing hips her daughter would develop, and said daughter weighed a good 9½ pounds at birth. That's a big baby. She struggled with breastfeeding but persevered and eventually, after a week, took me home to the house owned by her parents, Walter and Edna Jones.

I could not have been made more welcome. My mother was an only child, as I, given the horrors she'd gone through during my delivery, would also be. She determined never to have another child and endure such pain and fear again. I became the centre of everyone's attention. I was the ultimate chubby, healthy, strong-limbed bonny baby of whom the entire family was inordinately proud. It would be some years before my mother would bemoan the fact that I appeared to have inherited my father's powerful bone structure rather than her fine, delicate limbs. A nicely rounded baby was one thing, a somewhat hefty teenager was quite another.

I doubt maternal concerns have changed much during the subsequent sixty-nine years. I often see new young mothers around me proudly showing off their plump, dimpled offspring and explaining how he or she is so good and never fussy about eating whatever is put before him or her. Then come the mothers of the teenagers, deeply worried that their kids are too thin or too fat. The obsession with size and feeding begins at the very start of life and never seems to end.

In those early weeks after my mother and I returned home, there developed a problem. My mother began to notice an unpleasant smell, which no amount of bathing would dispel. She went back to the hospital for investigation and found a swab had been left inside her during the forceps delivery,

8

causing a terrible infection. Whilst she was being treated, her hungry baby had to be left at home and the breastfeeding, which she'd begun to master, was put on hold for a week. She expressed milk in the hospital to keep her supply going, whilst my grandmother took on the task of bottle-feeding me.

Grandma would often tell me what a hungry baby I'd been. How I would scream for more when a feed was finished, whether it was bottle or breast. I never seemed to have had enough. The feeding schedule, designed by Sir Truby King, a New Zealand health reformer and breastfeeding advocate, was, of course, extremely strict. A feed every four hours, regular as clockwork, and it should last for only ten minutes on each side during breastfeeding, or twenty minutes total for a bottle-feed. A crying baby must be left outside in the fresh air whatever the weather. Any further attention would spoil the child. The regime was popular, but also controversial.

I've often wondered if that week of separation from my mother disturbed the feeding pattern we'd established, to the detriment of both of us. For the rest of our lives together she often seemed resentful of the demands I made on her, and I seem to have learned early on what it was to be hungry and dissatisfied. When I fed my own two children I became very aware of how utterly unnatural and unsatisfactory the Truby King method must have been. For the early weeks and months of their lives my sons were virtually permanently attached to me, greedily consuming as much as they wanted for as long as they wanted. Neither of them grew up to have any kind of eating disorder and neither became fat.

For three years after I was born my father, mother and I lived with my grandparents. My father, working in a TV-repair shop and studying to become an electrical engineer, earned very little money. In 1953 a council estate was built behind the road where my grandparents lived and my parents moved in to one of the new houses. Now I had two homes where women ruled the roost and invested all their energy in caring for their households, making sure everything was immaculate, and doing their best to stave off the boredom they suffered. They were two highly intelligent and educated women whose days were filled with housework, shopping and the culinary arts.

Both had had to give up their jobs when they married. Grandma had worked in the accounts department of one of the big Yorkshire woollen mills; Mum had been a civil servant. The marriage bar, which banned married women from the Civil Service, ended in 1946, but it would take some time for employers to take the new rules on board and it was rare for a woman to consider it respectable to pursue a career *and* fulfil her domestic duties. Even in the twenty-first century, as we've seen often in cases of sex and gender discrimination or unequal pay, a change in the law does not always effect a change in custom and practice.

The entire family had, of course, suffered the deprivations of rationing during, and for a while after, the Second World War, although we had been lucky in that the men had not had to face the danger or aftermath of active conflict. My grandfather had been called up in 1918, just as the First World War was coming to a close, and my father in 1945. The Second World War had just finished. Grandpa's war was spent in the Royal Horse Artillery and seemed to involve a thoroughly enjoyable time galloping around London's parks with his fellow soldiers. Dad did spend some time abroad as a young engineer in Egypt and Italy, but he was working on the clean-up operations and, luckily for us all, saw no battles.

The wartime diet had meant a lot of hard work for women trying to cook well for their families when so much that helped make food delicious was not available. There'd been very little sugar, butter or meat, no sweets, not much fruit, and I remember clearly my father retching at the memory of the reconstituted-dried-egg sandwiches he'd had to take to school and then to work for his lunch.

Nevertheless, as far as healthy eating was concerned, the diet had probably been a pretty ideal one, as my grandfather was a wonderful gardener and grew a vast range of fruits and vegetables. He carried on providing the fruit and veg for the family and, as I became a toddler, the end of rationing for these two committed and traditional 1950s housewives was definitely something to celebrate. I would spend all the time I could in either my grandmother's kitchen or my mother's, sampling whatever goodies they had concocted. It's perhaps a trend to which we are now being persuaded to return as a new awareness of the importance of fresh fruit and vegetables and home cooking begins to be emphasized in place of processed ready meals. The only problem for the modern family is that great meals take time to shop for, prepare, eat and clear away. We often are tempted to take the easy way out.

Both my women loved to cook. My mother had not so much a kitchen shelf of cookery books as a library, and her bedtime reading was one or the other of what I guess I would now dub 'food porn'. The only author I really remember was Marguerite Patten, who'd been the popular wartime cook and was a star at teaching how to make the most of rationing. Post-war we didn't need her advice on how to cook whale – a thought that now sends shivers of horror down the spine. Her 1950s recipes were always good, solid traditional dishes such as fish pie, Irish stew, chocolate cake, treacle sponge pudding or a well-done roast of beef, all possible now the war was over and meat and ingredients for baking were back in the shops again. They all appeared regularly, along with her scones.

Fanny Craddock was a powerful influence on my mother's decorative instincts, with her fondness for a piping bag and vegetable colourings. I recall very clearly a lily-pond jelly. It was green, adorned with tinned pears in the shape of the flowers and sticks of green, sugary gelatin to make the reeds. The decoration was completed with swirls of piped whipped cream. I loved it and always took it to school for special events.

Of course, Elizabeth David's *A Book of Mediterranean Food* was published the year I was born and would change Britain's eating habits for ever as she introduced risotto and paella, polenta and spaghetti, aubergine and avocado, olive oil and garlic to the culinary mix. It was a bit of a problem sourcing ingredients that are now found everywhere, thanks to globalization. When I was a child the only olive oil you could get was in a tiny bottle at the chemist, intended for treating earache, apparently. How things have changed.

These days you can find a huge range of every possible ingredient necessary to follow David's beautiful recipes. Earlier today I counted twenty different olive oils on one shelf in my local supermarket. Some were virgin, some not, some were from Italy, some from Greece, some from Spain. None was particularly cheap, but they were flying off the shelves. My mother was keen to try David's recipes, but Dad was not happy. What he wanted was 'plain English food. None of this foreign muck.' Even my mother resisted garlic to the day she died. Whenever they came to stay I had to adjust my fondness for the Mediterranean diet.

My two cooks both devoted themselves to producing three wonderful meals every day and never ceased to make it plain at every available opportunity that their efforts in the kitchen were an expression of their undying love for and devotion to their families. We, in turn, were expected to show how grateful we were by never refusing to eat whatever was offered, always clearing the plates of the extremely generous portions we were given and always, always, always saying, 'That was delicious. Thank you so much!'

Breakfast at Grandma's was bacon, egg, mushrooms, tomatoes and fried bread. It was especially delicious at her house because she had an old kitchen range and frying was done over the open fire my grandfather had risen early to light. We were never short of coal for the purpose of cooking and heating the home. Grandpa's job was at the pit so a plentiful supply was part of his wages. Summer and winter the blaze glowed in the kitchen, and there was another fire just for heating in the sitting room.

I don't know why that method of frying made everything taste so spectacular, but what was cooked on the open fire was amazing. The bacon was crisp, the eggs were a little brown around the edges and had perfectly runny yolks. The fried bread was crunchy, and the tomatoes were soft and juicy and had the kind of rich flavour we hardly seem to get any more. The coal-fired method of baking and roasting produced equally extraordinary results, and the meat, bread, pies and Yorkshire puddings Grandma baked in the coal oven had to be tasted to be believed.

It's interesting that we've gone through a fast-food culture, which I have no doubt did us harm in terms of flavour and probably health-giving properties, as we've become so used to high levels of salt, fat and sugar, but there does seem to be a stirring of interest in going back to the traditional methods. Mary Berry has done a lot to promote the Aga, which doesn't have to be lit every day like an old coal oven, but Aga cooks swear by the enhanced flavour of anything prepared in such a way.

It certainly played a part in everything my grandma made. Her Yorkshire puddings rose up the pan and were crispy and light. Her scones, tarts and cakes were the best I've ever eaten. Well, that's not strictly true. I always thought her pastry couldn't be bettered, but one day on *Woman's Hour* Nigel Slater brought his apple pie and cream for me to try. I had to confess it was even better. Sorry, Gran.

In my family's own little house, the cooking method was a bit more modern. We had a gas cooker but no central heating, so it was a coal fire that heated the house and the water. There was no fridge, but a pantry, just as my grandmother had, so the production of daily menus really was a full-time job for Mum and Grandma. Shopping for food was performed each day after the other chores had been done. Cleaning and laundry were for the morning. Shopping in the afternoon. Ironing in the evening. Cooking at every other moment of the day.

As we lived close to each other the daily tasks were often shared. My mother had a washing machine. Grandma, up till then, had done all the laundry in a great tub outside the house with a manual mangle to squeeze out all the water. Then the clothes were hung out to dry, or positioned round the fire on a clothes horse if the weather was wet. She didn't want any 'new-fangled' appliances in her kitchen, so every Monday her dirty laundry was packed into a suitcase and brought to us. So many spectacular rows ensued as they tripped over one another in the kitchen and Grandma flooded the floor yet again. She never did quite master getting the pipe that emptied the twin tub into the sink, where it would drain away safely and without incident.

I would hide out of the way, often tucked into the hearth between the clothes horse and the fire with a good book and whatever treats Grandma had brought to keep me quiet and content. A simple bar of Cadbury's Dairy Milk with fruit and nuts, or maybe a Flake, would be enough to keep me happy from breakfast to lunch. On the rare occasions she had no treats to bring over, I'd be given sixpence and allowed to 'pop down the road' to the local shop to fill a bag with toffees, flying saucers and Sherbet Dib Dabs. Such 'treats' still exist, but seem to have become the focus of concerns about childhood obesity. There've been moves to make the portions smaller and the prices bigger in the 'war on sugar'.

In a report published in October 2019, 'The State of the World's Children', the United Nations Children's Fund (UNICEF) pointed to what it describes as 'food swamps' – communities oversaturated with unhealthy dining options – and says our poorest streets are littered with fast-food 'child magnets'. 'The UK retail food environment', it continues, 'encourages unhealthy foods consumption. Poorer areas also have more visible advertising for unhealthy foods than wealthier areas.' And it's not only the fast-food outlets that are causing problems. If a child pops into WHSmith to buy a pen, there's usually an offer of a huge bar of chocolate for £1, and at the cinema a vast bucket of popcorn costs only a few pence more than a smaller portion. It's a big worry in a country where rates of childhood obesity are among the highest in the developed world.

I saw my maternal grandmother just about every day. My paternal grandmother lived further away, but would always come for tea once a week. She shared Edna's delight at being able to bring sweet treats as rationing ended. I never would have dared to refuse any of their offerings. Not that I would have wanted to. I loved every kind of chocolate or biscuit that appeared – apart from Caramac, and I even ate that on one occasion so as not to appear ungrateful. Even the slightest hint that I was displeased with their gifts and didn't want to eat every scrap immediately would have engendered such hurt and disappointment that it would have been cruel not to scoff the lot at once.

The pair of them were very fat. They were also short and really as round as they were long, but no encouragement to go on a diet and lose weight had any impact on either of them. 'Don't be silly,' they would scoff to my mother. 'We're not bothered about being thin. What else is there for us to enjoy but nice food and sweets?' They didn't drink, they didn't smoke, they didn't go out much, and their primary entertainment was a little pile of romantic novels my mother and I would pick up for them from the library each week. And it has to be said that, fat as these two food lovers were, they were also extremely fit. They spent hours every day scrubbing and sweeping both inside and outside the house. The path to the front step had to be immaculate, and the step itself had to be scrubbed every morning and treated with a special polish called Red Cardinal. They were physically very hard workers. All a bit different from today's hard work – often sitting in front of a computer and nipping to the supermarket in the car.

I would often hear my mother muttering to herself that she just didn't understand how they 'could let themselves go' as she helped Grandma Edna struggle into the ample corset she wore whenever she left the house. It was a huge, boned pink thing and my mother would pull hard on the strings at the back to hold her in as tight as she could. It didn't seem to make much difference to the way my grandmother looked, and I was always pleased when she came home and, with a great sigh of relief, took it off. It was not comfortable to have a cuddle on her lap with the bones sticking into my tummy.

The pursuit of culinary brilliance and the expression of love through the food my mother and Grandma Edna created continued unabated throughout my childhood. After those wonderful breakfasts, which were dished up every day even after we moved to our own house, and with the cleaning, dusting and tidying up completed, I would have a good wash – we didn't have a shower, and a bath was only allowed three times a week, always before bed – my mother would plait my hair and dress me in nice clean clothes. A clean pair of knickers every day was insisted upon, 'in case you have an accident'. Mum would do her hair – she had it permed every six weeks and washed and blow-dried every Friday – put on her red lipstick – she never left the house without it – and, if it was a weekday, off we would go to the shops.

It was a good long walk down a steep hill into Worsborough village, where we knew every shopkeeper and had no trouble deciding what to buy where. There was the greengrocer whose produce we would need if Grandpa didn't have much ready in the garden. We only bought foods that were in season, but every conceivable vegetable and fruit was there to be had at the right time of year. Everything – potatoes, cabbage, carrots, oranges, the occasional banana – would go straight into Mum's shopping bag. There were no other bags, plastic or otherwise.

We'd then pop over to the butcher. During the week it might be mince for a shepherd's or cottage pie, maybe some lamb chops or some stewing steak or bits of chicken for a casserole. A beef, lamb or pork joint to roast, or a whole chicken, would only be bought on a Saturday from the top-class local farmer who brought such delights round in a van for the weekend.

The Co-op was a wonderful shop. It had scrubbed wooden floors covered in sawdust, mahogany counters and shelves, and a contraption where the money you paid was fired around the shop to the accounts department before being returned to the counter with the change. It all added to the fun and fascination of the place for a little girl. Where did the money go? How did the change come back? It was an early example of the mysteries of automation. We bought butter and lard there, cut from a huge chunk and wrapped in greaseproof paper. There was flour – self-raising and plain – soon to be mixed at home with the butter and lard and made into perfect pastry, or maybe one of my mother's signature chocolate cakes or treacle sponge puddings with home-made custard. No meal was considered complete without some sort of dessert.

Just thinking about it all makes me feel hungry and long to have the chance to experience what it was like all over again. No effort on my part, just sit down at the table and enjoy! Then again, there was an element of force-feeding about it. There was my mother's constant insistence that 'all must be eaten, nothing wasted'. Maybe not such happy memories after all, especially when I think of the bad habits for my future that were being laid down at home. The portions were huge, the courses non-negotiable, and there's no doubt I learned that eating a lot and having a very full tummy was a sign of a successful, comfortable and well-off family.

On the Co-op counter sat the huge, circular Cheddar cheese, Stilton or – Grandpa's favourite – Gorgonzola, ready to be cut with a great length of wire and weighed in beautiful, heavy, brass-weight scales. It too was wrapped in greaseproof paper. We also bought bags of tea – nothing fancy – and sometimes freshly ground coffee. The shop itself smelled exotic and exciting and, of course, not only was it reasonable in price, but you also collected dividends with every purchase. As a co-operative, you were entitled to a share of the profits – small amounts, but they mounted up as the weeks went on and resulted in a quite considerable saving.

Last stop was the sweet shop for a little treat to eat on the way home as a reward for having been a good girl. Sweets as rewards or expressions of love and affection was a running theme through my childhood. It's taken us an awfully long time to begin to realize what a potentially dangerous practice that is, but the taste for sugary foods, once established, never seems to go away. All my life I've had that famous line used in an advert for cream cakes, reputedly coined by Fay Weldon, running through my head: 'Naughty, but nice.' It's still there when I consider a chocolate eclair at the bakery. Always so hard to resist.

Children are easily seduced by such catchlines. No matter how old you are, the slogan 'finger lickin' good' is bound to come to mind as you pass a KFC or 'I'm lovin' it' as you're drawn towards a McDonald's. Coca-Cola is 'the real thing' and if you 'have a break' you'll 'have a KitKat'. The advertising companies know exactly what will stick in our heads and influence the choices we make and, as children between the ages of six and ten are said to spend around twenty-eight hours a week watching television, they're exposed to thousands of ads every year.

I doubt there's a parent in existence who hasn't experienced 'pester power', even though advertisers are told not to encourage kids to persuade their parents to buy them whatever they fancy. There's been much discussion about whether or not there should be stricter restrictions on advertising to children. So far there's an Advertising Standards Authority code, which requires marketers to check the audience profile of any media through which they plan to advertise. They are advised to avoid placing ads for foods or soft drinks that are high in fat, salt or sugar where more than 25 per cent of an audience is under the age of sixteen. It's all very difficult when parents, let alone the advertising industry, don't always know what children are watching, given the proliferation of TVs and electronic devices in children's own rooms.

Of course, when I was a little girl we never went to the bakery, except in a dire emergency. Bread – sometimes white, sometimes brown – was made at home, so we only needed to buy a loaf or maybe some biscuits if Mum had had a particularly hectic week. She made all the cakes and buns too, except the occasional custard slice, cream horn or chocolate eclair. Eclairs were Grandma's favourite and considered too fiddly to be home-made. They were special. The danger of 'treats' again!

The concept of the 'treat' is fascinating. What is it about us that falls for the hedonistic philosophy that lies behind that old Beverley Sisters song, suggesting that whatever gives you pleasure must be illegal or immoral or makes you fat? It's the 'naughty but nice' idea writ large. I suspect we feel, when we bite into the chocolate eclair, that we will love the sweetness of the chocolate, the texture of the pastry, the smoothness of the cream, but, because we have luxuriated in the pleasure, we must, surely, be punished. There's a part of all of us that wants to misbehave, even though we know we'll suffer as a result. It's why very few of us would elevate an apple to 'treat' status. It's nice, but it's not naughty!

Saturday afternoon at home was for going to town and for Mum, Grandma and me to go round Barnsley market – then the biggest and best open-air market in the country. You could find anything there – clothes, stockings, furniture, make-up, jewellery, crockery – all displayed to the crowds by master showmen, and, of course, my mother knew the stalls that had the freshest, most perfect fruit and vegetables. We'd go in on the two o'clock bus, spend an hour or so browsing the stalls and come only to the fruit and veg men and the fish stall at the end of the day.

My two, penny-pinching, 'look after the pence and the pounds will look after themselves' Yorkshire women would always arrive just before the stall holders were getting ready to pack up and would negotiate the most brilliant bargains. None of the market men wanted to be left with food that would perish over the weekend and we would come away well stocked up with the freshest of fresh food. For Saturday tea there'd be mussels from the fish stall, which Grandpa would prepare when we got home, or there might be a crab that would need to be hammered open at the tea table and eaten with freshly buttered bread and a salad. Sometimes there was a bit of halibut with parsley sauce – Grandma's favourite firm, creamy fish.

There's no doubt when it comes to the effort my family put into buying and cooking the finest-quality food they could afford. For a working-class family, with ambitions to rise beyond the pit and the council housing, it was an essential part of what needed to be shown to the world. My mother remembered taking an apple for playtime at the local village primary school she attended and other children would surround her, begging to be given the core she didn't want.

She told one story about a girl whose father would have an egg for breakfast and would smear a little yolk around his daughter's mouth to give the impression that she'd had one too. At one point, my mother – the winder's daughter, with a father who worked above ground and was consequently paid a little better than the men he wound up and down the mine shaft – was the only child in her class who had a pair of shoes.

When you've witnessed such poverty, you want to make sure that your family never suffers in such a way. You buy the best and hold to the belief that a family that eats together stays together. It wasn't acceptable for men to turn up late for their dinner because they'd spent what little time and money they had in the pub. Everyone had to be at the table on time. It was, though, the effort the women put into their jobs as housewives that made it all possible. These days, as men and women so frequently work outside the home, time is at a premium in a way it never was during my childhood.

Only one meal in the week was not home-made. Friday's special treat for lunch was fish and chips from the chippy round the corner. Mum would give me two bob and send me to bring back fish and chips twice, and some scraps. (Scraps are a Northern delicacy – the bits of loose batter that would be scraped up out of the fat after the fish was fried. They're delicious.) I could also buy a bottle of dandelion and burdock – my favourite pop, which I was allowed to have only once a week. The rest of the time I had to drink the juice of just one freshly squeezed orange, or water. One useful attempt at keeping sugar consumption down, I suppose.

Of course, there was no eating the food from the newspaper

in which it was wrapped. It had to be consumed correctly: on a plate at the dining table, and with a knife and fork, not fingers. I used to say we could save on the washing-up, but my mother would have none of it. I learned always to put the vinegar on first, then the salt, because vinegar washes off the salt if you put it on beforehand. All my life I've been asked in chippies if I want salt and vinegar and have always demanded, 'Yes, please – vinegar first, then salt.'

So many things learned in childhood are there for a lifetime. Some are good, some are bad, and the bad things are the hardest to shake off. I find it very tough, even now, to pass a chippy without sniffing the scent of frying, like a Bisto kid. It takes every ounce of willpower to stop myself going in.

The only meal provided by my mother that I hated was lunch on Monday – washday. Never one to waste a scrap of anything, she would slice what remained of the Sunday roast, fry it up with an onion and some gravy, and serve it with mashed potato and cabbage. It was disgusting. I wasn't really hungry – on account of Grandma's sweet treats, which I'd been scoffing all morning – so I would poke the lunch around my plate and say I felt sick and really couldn't eat it.

The idea of only eating when you were hungry was alien to my mother. 'You will eat every scrap,' she would say. 'I won't have a fussy eater.' No matter how little effort she'd put into the meal, she would be deeply insulted and upset at my refusal. I would watch the meat and gravy go cold. 'There's no pudding for you,' she would say. 'And you will eat that perfectly good plate of food, even if it's this evening, and you'll have it cold.' Several times I ended up eating icy, coagulated beef and onion for supper, and soon learned there was no point refusing anything she put before me. She had spent her time making it, I would have to eat it and clean the plate completely. Again, it's the fear of poverty, I believe, that made the obsession with plenty and hatred of waste so pronounced in my mother's generation.

The provision of a wholesome diet was another absolute fixation for the women, who saw it as their job to ensure that every member of the family was made strong and healthy and given pleasure by the constant appearance (well, except for washday lunch) of something really delicious to eat. And pleasure was central to the way meals were served and consumed. There was no grabbing something quickly in the kitchen. Hours of preparation went into virtually every meal. On the days I was at home or at Grandma's, I was expected to be the sous chef, learning the skills I would need as an adult when I would be required to 'find the way to a man's heart through his stomach'. Yes, my mother actually said that, and I doubt I'm alone in having heard those words over and over again. Friends of my era have the same memories of that hackneyed but familiar phrase that drove them crazy as they asked themselves, 'Is that it? Is that all I'm for, to clean and cook to keep a man happy?'

There was a stool in the kitchen, which is where I would sit up at the work surface and do my bit. Much of what my mother prepared was done from memory. She, like me, had sat alongside her mother and learned exactly how much flour, butter, lard and water needed to go into a perfect pastry mix. She did have recipes too. One or two of that huge collection of recipe books – most often Marguerite Patten – were always kept on her bedside table in the place where most of us would have a copy of whichever novel we are in the midst of, and there was an exercise book in the kitchen into which she would stick magazine cuttings with new ideas for the perfect chocolate cake, casserole or scone. She must have dreamed cakes, biscuits and curious things to do with jellies.

Mixing a chocolate cake is the first culinary art I remember being taught. Mum would measure the flour, sugar, cocoa and butter into a big mixing bowl. I would cream everything together with a wooden spoon for ages until it was completely smooth and it was time to add the egg. More creaming, lifting the mixture up and down to introduce as much air as possible and then, when she said I had done enough, I would butter the cake tin and she would pour the mixture into it, then pop it into the oven and give permission for my treat: I could lick whatever remained in the bowl, and would scrape out every scrap of raw mixture with my fingers. I loved it; and then came the inimitably delicious smell of a chocolate cake baking in the oven. The whole kitchen held the sweet scent of our efforts every single day.

Even when my hands were tiny I was expected to wash them, cool them under the cold tap and rub the flour and fat together to the consistency of breadcrumbs in preparation for making pastry. Mum would add the cold water, worried that my hand might slip and I would make the mixture too sloppy. She would bind it all together and give me the job of sprinkling flour on to the worktop and carefully rolling out the pastry to the right thickness. She would take the correct amount for an apple pie and I would roll again, cutting lots of small pastry linings ready to make jam tarts.

I would butter the tart tins so the pastry wouldn't stick, pop just the right amount of jam into each one and leave the actual baking to my mother. I was a teenager before I was allowed to go anywhere near a hot oven. I looked forward so much to my father coming home and eating those tarts. Yes, I was falling into the trap of finding the way to a man's heart through his stomach, but I adored my father and did learn there could be great pleasure in the careful preparation of good food and seeing someone you love enjoy it.

Pleasure and the gathering of a family around a table seems often to be something so many of us have lost in the twenty-first century, but it was such an important part of my childhood. Meals were never consumed in a hurry and always had an air of formality about them. Whether we ate at my grandmother's or at our own house, the kitchen table had to be set for breakfast, which meant getting up in good time, washing, dressing and sitting down to eat and talk about whatever was planned for the day.

When it came to lunch or dinner, the table in the dining room had to be laid for however many people would be sitting down. A clean tablecloth, beautifully crisp and ironed, was placed over an old blanket, designed to protect the wood beneath from any heat from plates or serving dishes. Knives, forks, spoons, glasses, a cruet and serviettes were placed in their correct positions and everyone sat down, waiting to be served by the chief cook – either Grandma or Mum. We would all sit together at my house. No elbows on the table. Immaculate table manners. No reading. Mealtimes were for chatting, joking and setting the world to rights.

There was only one exception to these very strict rules. If we were eating at Grandma's she was allowed to get up and down from the table whenever she chose. To be honest, I hardly remember her sitting down at all. She was so anxious that everyone else should have a perfect serving of the food she'd cooked that she would often eat her own portion standing in the kitchen as she stirred the custard or checked that the sponge pudding would be ready at exactly the right time.

After we'd been served she would hover at the edge of the table like an anxious housemaid or butler, ready to whisk away any empty plate and rush it off to the kitchen. She couldn't bear her kitchen to be in a mess and certainly didn't expect her husband or any other member of the family to help with the washing-up. Nevertheless, I loved to eat at her home. My mother was a great cook and somewhat more experimental than my grandmother, but Grandma Edna, as described by her husband, had a touch of magic about her culinary skills. 'She waves her wand over everything,' he would say, and there's no doubt the magic was there in her buttery, crumbly, melt-in-the-mouth pastry; crisp, delicate Yorkshire puddings; and the lightest, fluffiest Victoria sponge ever made.

Even what she referred to as her 'Yorkshire peasant dishes' were tastier than anything I've ever eaten. The most memorable was a corned-beef hash which she made with a tin of corned beef, cubed potatoes, carrots, onions and her own home-made stock. She added pearl barley and lentils to bulk it out and served beetroot, grown by my grandfather, and boiled and pickled by her, as a side dish. It came out as a steaming stew, served in the hollow of a perfect Yorkshire pudding. It was my favourite Wednesday-evening supper.

I always stayed at her house on Wednesday and Saturday evenings – to give my parents some time to go out together, I suppose. The only thing Grandpa made, apart from the mussels he would clean and boil for Saturday tea, were chips for supper late on Saturday night before bedtime. He sliced the potatoes nice and thin with a special sharp knife he'd made himself, heated the lard in a chip pan over the open fire in the kitchen, and out they came – perfectly brown, a little crisp on the outside, soft on the inside, vinegar first and salt second. The best chips ever. These memories are so clear and so much at the forefront of everything I recall from my childhood. Those chips were so good I can still taste them!

The interesting thing about the impact all this wonderful food had on me is that I never got fat and I never thought about whether I was over- or underfed, or ought to be worrying about myself. The only slightly dark hint about the risk of getting fat was my mother's constant concern about my grandmother and how she had 'let herself go'. Yes, I was a well-rounded, chubby baby, but as I grew and began to move around, the plumpness disappeared. Until my early teens I was strong and solid and amazingly healthy without a scrap of fat anywhere on my body.

Admittedly I got plenty of exercise. We had no car until Dad bought a van for work, and even then it was rarely available for me to take advantage of. Dad worked incredibly long hours and Mum couldn't drive. Our trips to the village shops necessitated a good long walk down the hill and an arduous stretch back up it to get home, carrying heavy bags full of shopping. When we went to Barnsley market it was a walk to the bus stop and then a good walk around town. When I started school there was no form of transport apart from the same bus into town and a long walk to the school, or later, as I grew older, the bike.

Even though we lived on a council estate there was plenty of unspoiled countryside around us. My best friend, John from next door, and I would spend every moment we could walking in the woods with a picnic, climbing trees, roller-skating down the street outside the house or going off for the afternoon on our bikes.

The World Health Organization says children and youths from five to seventeen should have sixty minutes of moderate to vigorous physical activity every day. We know from scientific research that the kind of food we consume plays more of a role in the development of obesity than the amount of exercise we do, but, as childhood obesity rates continue to rise, we must bear in mind that a diet of poor, processed food, accompanied by sweet fizzy drinks, combined with a car culture, the loss of school playing fields, the habit of online gaming rather than playing outdoors and parents' fears of letting children out of our sight, must be having a damaging influence on children's physical and mental health.

I had no interest in any form of sport. The cricket and football played by the boys and the rounders the girls seemed to enjoy bored me to tears. Dad, who loved badminton and tennis, tried to get me to join him, but gave up when he realized I was genuinely lacking the hand–eye coordination required to hit a shuttlecock or a ball. It was my grandfather who sparked a sporting passion in me that lasted for a very long time.

As a young man, my grandfather's best friend at work happened to be the farrier who looked after the pit ponies. They received their call-up papers at the same time, at the end of the First World War. 'Well,' said Grandpa, 'I suppose we'd better volunteer for t'infantry.' 'No chance,' said his friend. 'I'm not walkin' abart. We'll go into t'cavalry.' 'Can't do that,' said Grandpa. 'I don't know 'ow to ride a 'orse.' 'Ee, don't worry, lad, they'll bloody teach you!'

And that's how my grandfather became an expert horseman. When I was only two years old, as the pit ponies were made redundant, thanks to automation, Grandpa's friend's daughter applied to take over the pit stables that had been used to give the ponies R and R and the field belonging to the National Coal Board so that she could use the ponies to start a riding school. They agreed. Grandpa took me there on the opening day, sat me on a bay pony called Captain and taught me to ride. I had found my sport and only gave it up in my fifties after a hip replacement made me a little more cautious than I'd ever been before about falling off and coming a cropper.

So there was plenty of exercise to keep me fit, but it's my recent research into the science of how the body copes with copious amounts of food that has made me wonder if it was not the quality of the food I ate that really made the difference to my weight; perhaps a child growing up today would have the same results. In his book *The Diet Myth*, Tim Spector, Professor of Genetic Epidemiology at King's College London, introduced me to the importance of the microbiome.

The microbiome is the genetic material of all the millions of microbes – bacteria, fungi, protozoa and viruses – that live on and inside the human body. The gut microbiome plays a very important role in our health by helping to control digestion and benefitting our immune system. An imbalance of unhealthy and healthy microbes in the intestines may contribute to weight gain, high blood sugar and high 'bad' cholesterol.

Alongside an analysis of which fats, proteins and carbo-hydrates are good and which are not so good – something we spend a lot of time thinking about these days – Professor Spector slips in this fascinating piece of information. He says the 'fat is deadly' message, which has been so common in recent years, has caused diets to change for the worse. The exclusion of saturated fats has reduced the diversity of foods we eat and our intake of many nutrients. The French, he says, eat more saturated fat – butter and cheese, for example – than Anglo-Saxons. They have less heart trouble than people in the UK and live longer than Americans.

The healthier habits of southerners in France is, he says, the answer. The French in general enjoy a regular diet full of living things, and in this category he includes cheese, wine and yogurt, which teem with living microbes. Cheese, he explains – not the processed kind – helps maintain the natural healthy microbiome. He also says, 'If you see natural food, for instance the bacteria in blue cheese, as dangerous and industrial food as healthy, you're losing much of what your body needs.'

Spector asks a crucial question. Could microbes be the new fat-eaters? He cautions against probiotics included in yogurts. Some commercial yogurt brands, he says, over-emphasize the benefits because they include sugar, which stops bacteria growing. He recommends consuming a wide range of beneficial bacteria and microbe-fertilizers rather than relying on a few species of bacteria that are added commercially.

Looking back to my childhood diet, I am struck by the extent to which it fits what Professor Spector advises. It was never processed food. It included a vast range of fresh fruits and vegetables, often grown, including the tomatoes, in my grandfather's garden, washed to get the soil off but then eaten raw or lightly cooked. As for cooking, Grandma would insist we drank the water in which the veg – which might be cabbage or even nettles – had been boiled to 'make sure you get the vitamins and goodness'. There must have been lots of healthy microbes from the environment in there.

The fats my family used were lard and butter. Margarine and processed cooking oils came much later. We never drank red wine, but there was occasional home-made apple cider or ginger beer, which must have teemed with microbes. Then there's the cheese. It was never processed, and let me remind you that Grandpa's favourite – and mine – was Gorgonzola. He liked it best when it stank to high heaven and 'threatened to walk off the plate'! A mass of healthy bacteria!

Without any knowledge of the latest food science, sixty years ago my family instinctively provided what Professor Spector, in 2015, says quite clearly is a good diet. And it's worth pointing out that, despite being unquestionably fat, neither Grandma nor any other member of the family ever developed that common disease of the modern era: type 2 diabetes.

'Fat for most is not the villain. Saturated fat in yogurt and cheese is likely to be beneficial, providing it's real, contains living microbes and isn't over processed or full of other unwanted chemicals or sweeteners,' Spector writes.

His most recent research – *The Diet Myth* published in 2015 and his foreword to *The Healthy Gut Handbook* in 2017 – has brought him to warn women to avoid Caesarean sections if they possibly can, as an infant's time passing through the birth canal is the best thing ever for the microbiome. Given the amount of time I spent there before I was finally dragged out by the forceps, I must have had the best microbial start in life.

Now to figure out where such an auspicious beginning went so wrong.

2

Unhealthy Eating

I was not a fat teenager, but I certainly didn't fit in with the fashion of the time. If Marilyn Monroe had stayed in style I would probably have been considered more or less OK. As Dad often said, what a pity it was that women like her and Jane Russell – women 'with a bit of meat on them' – seemed no longer to be attractive. Everyone wanted to look like Twiggy – straight up and down, flat-chested and skinny as can be.

Of course that's exactly what I wanted to be. I bought all the fashion magazines, pored over the pictures of Twiggy and Jean Shrimpton, and hoped I too would look stunning with a Vidal Sassoon bobbed haircut, the shortest of short skirts, long, slender legs and great big, seductive, fluttery eyes. There wasn't much hope for a teenager from Yorkshire to take herself down to London and shop in Mary Quant's boutique in Chelsea, but good old Barnsley market did a great line in copies that were much more affordable than the King's Road or Biba.

It was from this cultural moment when I was around the age of fourteen that I can date my increasing anxiety about my strong, big body. 'Don't worry, love,' my mother would say, 'you're not fat, you're just big-boned.' That reference to my inheritance of my father's hefty frame again. All the more upsetting coming from a mother who prided herself on her slender wrists and ankles and the fact that when they married Dad could span her then-tiny waist with his hands. She was not a picky eater and she did put on a little weight as she headed towards middle age, but the delicate bones, the slender legs and wrists, never changed. I guess she was lucky in the genes she inherited. Her father had a fine bone structure and never became fat in the way my grandmother did.

It wasn't only my mother who made me feel inadequate. One boyfriend with whom I went swimming – the only other sport apart from riding at which I was any good – told me I had great legs. 'Just like a gladiator,' he laughed. He didn't last long.

When I look back on those teenage years I realize that, even though I was no Twiggy, I was a perfectly fit and healthy young woman. I grew to 5 feet 7 inches and never weighed more than 9 stone despite the constant droning on at home about feeding me up. My father's job took him abroad for long periods as I reached my teenage years and my mother would divide her time between us. Sometimes, when my mother went with him, I would live with my grandparents and enjoy exactly the same fresh and varied diet I'd had throughout my childhood.

I stayed slim, despite the constant flow of massive meals, and managed to wear the short, short skirts that we all changed into once our school uniform was dropped on to the bedroom floor and we could get ready to go out. I do, though, remember the very short leather mini becoming a little tight around the waist at one point before my mother came home and took control of my diet. I can only blame my grandmother – her cakes, scones, chocolate treats and spectacular Yorkshire puddings – for the few extra pounds I seemed to gain.

34

I must have been around fifteen years old when my mother came home to stay for a long period and I steadfastly refused her constant encouragement to 'wear a Playtex girdle, love, it'll keep your tummy nice and flat'. This was the mid-sixties and the feminist ideologies that would emerge later in the decade had not yet begun to encourage the abandonment of the bra, but no self-respecting girl in the midst of the sexual revolution would be seen wearing what was essentially a rubber corset.

Nevertheless, I have no doubt our conversations about 'keeping my tummy nice and flat' had a profound influence on my confidence in my own body. We've learned that fat shaming our children by criticizing their weight, their size or the amount they eat is dangerous as it can lead to further overeating and obesity, or its opposite – anorexia. In my case it engendered a constant sense of anxiety that I just didn't look 'good enough'.

I put my trust in my horse riding and games at school to keep my muscles toned, and underwear was carefully chosen and as skimpy as possible. After all, we had to wear baggy grey knickers at school – the rules around uniform were strict and the grey pants couldn't be hidden. They were on show during gym and were absolutely regulation. In our own time, out of school, it was a lacy bra, pretty pants, tights and a mini. We were beginning to be interested in boys, but had no intention of them ever seeing our lovely undies. The fear of pregnancy was far too great for us to risk even the lightest of petting.

The subtle changes in my weight, and indeed my mother's, began soon after she, with my encouragement, got a job. She'd been desperately concerned about the friends and neighbours who, she said, would think she'd had to get one because Daddy couldn't afford to keep us. Patently that was not the case. Dad was working hard and doing well as an electrical engineer but, for once, she took my advice and my reassurance that there was absolutely nothing wrong with a woman going out to work and earning her own money. It was no reflection on the respectability of the family.

It meant, though, that she became a little less assiduous about her shopping for fresh and varied ingredients, and her greater exposure to the outside world introduced her to the new trends the food industry was bringing to the shops. It was my first experience of that terrible feminist dilemma – it's women who're generally expected to provide the food for the family, but a woman who goes out to work has less time for shopping and cooking, so families often eat less well if both parents work outside the home. It's taking far longer than it should for mothers and fathers to acknowledge that taking care of a family is a joint responsibility.

Of course, my mother still made her weekend trips to the market for fresh fruit and veg, and her selection of meat was always of the best quality, but, as a working woman, she didn't have the time to spend slaving over a hot stove, creating gourmet menus, and, just as I had been genning up on fashion in the magazines, she had been reading about new and processed foods.

I, of course, was all for embracing the new. I even remember encouraging her to stop bothering with baking her own bread – wholemeal and delicious – and instead to start buying white sliced like everybody else was, all wrapped up in plasticky paper. I recall telling her it would be so much easier not to have to keep slicing the bread ourselves and, according to the manufacturers' adverts, it would last longer. Of course it did – it was full of preservatives. There was still lots of cooking to be done, and baking of cakes and pastries at the weekend, but things began to change significantly as the industrialization of food began to take a hold.

We'd always used butter and lard as our fats for frying and baking. Then Mum read that saturated animal fats were fattening and very, very bad for you. The advice about what's healthy and what's not seems to be changing constantly and now much of what was beginning to be sold as the best in the mid-sixties is the very opposite. But then advice can change almost on a daily basis. One moment in 2019 sausages, bacon and steak were carcinogenic; the next, another study said they're fine. It's more than confusing.

In my mother's home, suddenly margarine came into the house and products called Spry and Crisp 'n Dry, heavily marketed as better for your health, replaced everything that had gone before. I'm part of a generation that began to be raised on margarines and cooking oils, all of which were used both at home and in cakes, pastries, biscuits and burgers we bought in the shops. Now it's all about olive oil – the more virgin the better.

The composition of olive oil depends on the cultivar, the altitude at which the olives were grown, the time at which they were harvested and the process by which the oil was extracted. Extra-virgin is the most expensive form of the product and is best used for dipping and salad dressings. It doesn't fare well during cooking as it burns too easily, spoiling its flavour. Cheaper, refined olive oil is best for frying. I did try to introduce it to my mother and father. They hated the taste of it almost as much as they loathed garlic! I love it.

Where the local chippy had fried items in saturated animal

fat, which hadn't had all its goodness processed out of it, the new Wimpy bars – the first fast-food outlets, which became so popular, serving watery cappuccino, burgers in a bun and chips – were using trans fats. Now, in the twenty-first century, these are classed as dangerous to health. There are some naturally occurring trans fats in meats and milk, but it's in the manufactured ones, when hydrogen is added to liquid vegetable oils in order to make them more solid, where the danger lies. They've been found to raise levels of 'bad' LDL cholesterol and contribute to an increased risk of heart disease and stroke.

The National Institute for Health and Care Excellence (NICE) has asked for industrially manufactured trans fats to be banned and said their exclusion from people's diet would prevent 40,000 deaths a year. The amount of these fats found in food in the twenty-first century has been reduced significantly, but they're still to be found in cheap fried and processed items, which can form a large part of people's food intake, particularly when you consider the information in that recent UNICEF report, where concerns were expressed about how children from low-income families were being seduced by what they called 'food swamps'.

Professor Tim Spector warns that such foods put children at risk of developing fatty livers and other health concerns, and will lead inevitably to what he calls the Junk Food Obesity Storm. In the UK, he says, one-third of children under the age of ten eat junk food every day. In the US, 1 in 3 people eats in a fast-food restaurant daily. Typically, excessive amounts of fat, sugar and salt in foods are used to tickle the taste buds, but never really satisfy the appetite. They inhibit the growth of bacteria in the food and increase its shelf life, but for the consumer they mean too much fat, too many calories and chemicals, and a lack of fibre. There's a lack of diversity in such a diet, which is based on nothing but corn, wheat, soy, sugar, salt and meat, and, according to Spector, it's crisps, chips and processed meat that lead to the greatest increases in weight.

Of course, junk food is cheap, an easy choice and full of flavour. I've been there so many times. That sudden urge as you pass a McDonald's or a Burger King to taste that sweet, sugary flavour and then that sense of revulsion that the chips don't taste like fried potatoes at all and the burger is so greasy it leaves an unpleasant taste in your mouth. But it was convenient, it filled a hungry hole for a short time and the next time you're passing, that sweet addiction will kick in again.

Mum's trust in the food industry was total. For the first time, alongside the white sliced bread and margarine, and the cakes and biscuits bought in the shops, came ready meals, which we convinced ourselves were nutritious and adventurous. How we could have thought a Vesta beef curry should be classified as tasty food I can't imagine, but we did. We ate these meals because they were fancy and foreign and we were keen to widen our experience of other culinary cultures. We somehow managed to ignore the fact that they tasted revolting and the rice that came with the artificially flavoured curry sauce was the palest white and bland.

Similarly we'd buy Chinese food from the takeaways that were springing up. Our favourite dish was sweet and sour pork. I dread to think how much sugar was used to make it so sweet. Then came pizzas. Just white bread, really, but we convinced ourselves they were good for us because they had tomato purée and cheese on them. Of course, the cheese was processed. It was doing nothing for our microbial health. We'd swapped real food for an illusion.

I suspect everything we bought to make life easier was loaded with trans fats, salt and sugar. We'd always had sugar, of course, in cakes and puddings, but it had never gone into a chicken stew or a corned-beef hash. And it went into even the savoury ready meals. As the industrialization of food manufacturing and powerful advertising convinced us these meals would change the life of the overworked housewife or woman who worked outside the home, by taking the effort out of shopping and cooking and delighting us with wonderful flavours, ingredients that were not in themselves all bad were making their way on to our plates in far greater quantities than were good for our health. Convenience foods were inexpensive and easy. And they were fattening.

In my household, neither my mother nor I became remotely obese, but Mum, who was heading towards her forties, threatened by middle-age spread and living a much more sedentary lifestyle now she was at work all day, began to read about the new dieting revolution and a company called Weight Watchers. The idea had begun in 1961, pioneered by a New York housewife called Jean Nidetch. She'd been overweight all her life and at the age of thirty-eight she weighed in at 214 pounds, or 15½ stone. She had tried pills, hypnosis and numerous faddy diets, had lost weight and then inevitably regained it. It's what happens to so many of us. We gain weight, we lose it on a diet, we begin to eat 'normally' when we've dropped a few pounds, up it goes again, and we often end up weighing more than before we began the diet. In desperation, Nidetch joined up for a free ten-week weight-loss programme sponsored by the New York City Board of Health's obesity clinic.

The diet followed was developed in the 1950s by Dr Norman Jolliffe, head of the board's Bureau of Nutrition. Followers were ordered never to skip meals, eat fish five times a week, eat two pieces of bread a day and drink two glasses of skimmed milk. Liver once a week was included, along with plenty of fruit and vegetables. Alcohol was prohibited, as were sweets and fatty foods. Strict portion control was essential, so every item to be consumed had to be weighed.

Nidetch lost just over a stone in the ten weeks, but she found it very hard to resist her favourite cookies. She decided to avoid the meetings arranged for the programme, finding the group leaders too domineering, and set up her own weekly support group in her apartment. It began with six other women. Within two months it had grown to forty and it was their intention to offer each other support and share stories and ideas. The meetings included a weekly weigh-in and Nidetch invented a reward system so that women who achieved their milestones would win prizes. By October 1962 Nidetch had achieved her target of 142 pounds, or 14 stone 2 pounds. She claimed never to weigh more than 15 stone again.

The message spread quickly and Nidetch began to coach groups in other neighbourhoods. One couple, Al and Felice Lippert, were very keen to make their group a success. They lost weight and Al, a businessman in the garment industry, persuaded Nidetch to make a business out of her idea. Weight Watchers Inc. was launched in Queens in 1963. The first official meeting attracted four hundred attendants. Lippert franchised the company in 1964. Graduates from the programme were offered the right to use the name and methods for an inexpensive franchise fee, and 10 per cent of their gross earnings were paid to the parent company. By 1967, the company was international and my mother thought it would be a jolly good idea if we were to join up. I wasn't particularly overweight at the time, but I still had dreams of looking like Twiggy. I went along with my mother's suggestion, or should I say pressure, to keep her company. She was a hard woman to resist.

Our group back then was led by a fierce and rather bullying woman who claimed to have gone from 18 stone to 9 stone as a result of following the Weight Watchers programme. We were told every week exactly what foods we were allowed to consume and reminded of what was banned. Weighing scales, she said, would be our best friends – the ones in the kitchen on which we would weigh our food portions and the ones in the bathroom on which we would weigh ourselves.

I've never endured such a miserable and humiliating time in my life. Food ceased to be a pleasurable experience as my mother carefully measured every item that would make its way to our plate. She was also persuaded to buy Weight Watchers' products. I dread to think what was in the soups and tasteless concoctions she brought home, but they were revolting. Enough to make you want to stop eating altogether or, at least, head for a sneaky biscuit or cake to remind you that things could taste good.

The weekly weigh-in was appalling. My mother seemed to be quite successful. She always did have rather an iron will and her weight gain had never been considerable. I neither lost nor gained, probably due to the fact that, although my diet was under Mum's strict control at home, I ate what I liked for school lunches. Meat and potato pie and cherry custard tart were favourites at school and I never restricted myself when it came to them.

The other women and some men who made up our group were much fatter than Mum and I were and I watched them shake as they walked towards the scales and burst into tears as they found they hadn't lost but gained. 'No prize for you,' the group leader would shout. 'You should be ashamed of yourself.' And the gainers were indeed ashamed and deeply unhappy, and as we all left the hall there was quite a bit of mumbling about popping to the chippy or maybe nipping into the pub to seek solace.

I don't know if this was how all Weight Watchers sessions were run in the early days, but the company grew and grew. However, Mum and I didn't last very long. She had often been Dieter of the Week and would show off to her friends about the one or two lost pounds for which she had been highly praised, but I think we both became heartily sick of spending so much time being obsessed with weighing everything we ate and never feeling we were really allowed to enjoy our food. We gave up after a few months. I think it had really saddened us to see so many truly obese people struggling so hard to lose weight. It looked to us as though they weren't supported by membership of the group; instead, they were constantly humiliated. But perhaps it was just us who saw it this way.

It's interesting that the company was taken over by Heinz in 1978, netting the founders $72 million. Lippert remained chairman and Nidetch retained her role as consultant, but I remember even then, before I had researched and begun to understand the science behind how each individual body handles weight gain and weight loss – of that, more later – thinking what a brilliant business model it seemed to be. Heinz produced baked beans and tomato ketchup – favourites among children and young people – which were loaded with sugar. Reduced-salt and -sugar varieties are a relatively recent introduction. So in theory they could sell you the sweet things that contributed to making you fat, then charge you a fee to attend Weight Watchers where you could try to lose what you'd put on. I'll never know if this was really their thinking – Heinz no longer owns Weight Watchers in any event, and hasn't done for some time – but it appeared a plausible strategy to me, at least.

It was some time after my teenage years that I encountered Nancy Roberts, a New York journalist whose father had been a famous radio presenter. Her mother was a well-known cartoonist who invented Betty Boop and her brother was the actor Tony Roberts, who often played Woody Allen's best friend in films, such as in *Annie Hall*. Nancy lived in a tiny flat in Central London with her partner Uwe, a German banker, and was one of the warmest, funniest, most energetic and fattest women I've ever known.

It was my friendship with Nancy that began my education in the politics of fatness and food. Nancy had always been fat – as a little girl and as a teenager – unlike her parents and her brother. From her earliest years, her mother had taken her to see every diet doctor in New York and she had been forced into every slimming regime known to man, including being given pills to suppress her appetite. She would, she told me, lose weight, then put it all back on and then some. As a young woman, safely ensconced in London, away from her mother's constant criticism about her size, she would dread the transatlantic phone calls from her. 'As soon as I hear her voice,' she said, 'I reach immediately for one, two, even three bars of chocolate.'

Nancy spread her message that we should all learn to like ourselves, regardless of our size, in regular appearances on a phone-in she ran on Talk Radio. She would always say, 'I'm not a doctor,' but she was a listening ear and a comforting voice, giving advice to people who phoned up with deep anxiety about the way they looked. As a result she wrote a book called *Breaking All the Rules: Looking Good and Feeling Great No Matter What Your Size*. To her credit, she practised what she preached, enjoying her food, having an active relationship with her partner and always looking outstandingly stylish.

Nancy became a member of a theatre group called Spare Tyre and in 1979, inspired by Susie Orbach's book *Fat Is a Feminist Issue*, they produced a play called *Baring the Weight*. Susie had grown up in London but had spent much of her time in the US and, as a psychotherapist, had begun to talk to a lot of women who suffered from eating disorders. It was the constant availability of food that tormented so many wives and mothers, the responsibility these women felt for feeding their families, and the temptation to alleviate boredom by comfort eating that prompted Susie to write the book she hoped would change the world.

Her aim was to help women to understand their own bodies and their appetites, feel proud of who they were, even if they didn't fit the slender ideal, and to learn to, as she put it, 'Listen to your appetite. When you're hungry, and by that I mean hungry, not starving, eat, and when your appetite tells you you're full, stop.' It's a totally sensible idea, but for years and years I joked to myself that my appetite was the only subject on which I was profoundly deaf.

The Orbach psychology is not dissimilar to another put forward recently, in 2018, forty years after *Fat Is a Feminist Issue*. Called *Eat It Anyway: Fight the Food Fads, Beat Anxiety and Eat in Peace*, it's written by two young women, Eve Simmons and Laura Dennison, both of whom – as is still so common among young people who find themselves constantly under the surveillance of followers on social-media sites such as Instagram and Facebook – had suffered from bulimia and anorexia, and had learned to stamp out the kind of guilt they had associated with eating and putting on weight.

The two women have been remarkably frank about their own struggles and are anxious to point out in their book that throughout history food has never been a simple matter. As Laura explains, she recalls a carefree time in her life when she and her boyfriend would often go out to dinner together. It had been about much more than simply satisfying their hunger. It had been about romance, adventure and experimentation, but her eating disorder ended those pleasures.

'To this day,' she writes, 'that euphoric sense of food free-dom and bewildering excitement is yet to return. I pick what I fancy, but I'm not salivating at the thought of my incoming pudding, nor can I ever quite pluck up the courage to order something totally obscure on the off chance that I might like it. To those who relate to the screaming sense of enchantment that food choices elicit, I beg you to harness it, cherish it and choose unwisely – with your eyes, stomach and whichever part of your body is intrigued by what garlic-basted snails may taste like.'

Eve and Laura's stated intention that we should all relearn the sheer pleasure of eating, without being constantly obsessed with our waistlines or what constitutes 'healthy eating', pretty much chimes with what Nancy Roberts was saying all those years ago. *Baring the Weight* was publicized as being about 'self-image, eating disorders and how the rotten dieting indus-try was ruining our lives'.

Watching the play first introduced me to the idea that those of us who lose weight through dieting will regain the weight and most probably get even fatter than we were before the diet. The science that backs up this claim came much later, and we'll explore that in due course. But even early on, Weight Watchers came in for criticism, notably for that high rate of recidivism, where a successful slimmer regains the weight they have lost and comes back to the programme to begin again.

The company still operates; it recently changed its name from Weight Watchers to WW and claims to have revolution-ized its programme. There's still a points system to guide you towards the 'right' foods and away from the 'wrong' ones, a detailed description of the kind of physical activity you should be involved in, and access to mindfulness exercises. Interest-ingly, in 2012, before the rebrand, Zoe Hellman, Head of Health Policy for Weight Watchers, told the All Party Parliamentary Group on Body Image that they advocate a 5–10 per cent weight loss. It seems an odd statement to make when their products and services appear to me to be targeted at people who think they have so much more weight to lose. In my case, at my heaviest – 24 stone – I believed a 50 per cent loss was what I needed.

The company experienced ups and downs in its popularity as other weight-loss programmes and diets came on the scene, but enjoyed a boost when, in 2015, Oprah Winfrey, the Ameri-can broadcaster and writer who has struggled with her weight for decades, made the news by buying a 10 per cent stake in it. Stock prices more than doubled by the end of the day on which the announcement was made. Renewed interest in Weight Watchers and Slimming World was also brought about in 2019 after the phenomenal success of a book called *Pinch of Nom*, said to contain recipes that fit the low-calorie dietary rules of both programmes without swearing allegiance to any one diet plan. The book was authored by two very overweight women, Kate Allinson and Kay Featherstone, who published a hundred slimming recipes for home cooking. They explained they were keen to lose weight in a way that didn't feel as if they were punishing themselves.

It is, unquestionably, a diet book, using the same tricks that are found in Weight Watchers and Slimming World. The two professional cooks, who had run a restaurant in the Wirral, recommend using onion or garlic granules in soups and stews to keep any fuss and cost to a minimum, and advocate the use of low-calorie ingredients such as sweeteners, fat-free yogurts, reduced-fat spreads, low-fat cheese and skinless chicken. They have been together for fourteen years, say they are not skinny minnies or poster girls, and despite losing 14 stone between them over the course of a year admit they still have a long way to go. Their blog is the most visited in the UK and the book has shot to the top of the culinary bestseller lists.

It's not been unusual for Oprah Winfrey to promote ideas about wellness, and her battles with weight loss and weight gain are legendary. Business analysts were convinced that her investment in and endorsement of the company, and her abil-ity to promote the Weight Watchers programme, would be a boon, particularly as it seemed that this time she was invest-ing in what was always promoted as a sound, scientifically proven weight-loss method. A number of studies have shown that Weight Watchers, together with other popular diets – Atkins, Zone and South Beach – did indeed lead to an average loss of 10 pounds a year for those who followed the plan religiously.

However, as Traci Mann, Professor of Social and Health Psychology at the University of Minnesota and the author of

Secrets from the Eating Lab: The Science of Weight Loss, the Myth of Willpower and Why You Should Never Diet Again, wrote, 'Winfrey's venture is, in fact, a brilliant investment, although not necessarily for the reason she thinks. It's brilliant not because Weight Watchers works, but because it doesn't. It's the perfect business model. People give Weight Watchers the credit when they lose weight. Then they regain the weight and blame themselves. This sets them up to join Weight Watchers again. And they do.'

According to Professor Mann, the company has talked about this model to its shareholders. She saw a copy of its 2001 business plan, which said its membership 'have demonstrated a consistent pattern of repeat enrolment over a number of years'. In an interview for a 2013 documentary, *The Men Who Made Us Thin*, the former finance director of the company, Richard Samber, who was in place from 1968 to 1993, explained that the reason the business was so successful was because the majority of customers regained the weight they had lost. 'That's where your business comes from,' he said.

Weight Watchers denied this claim, arguing that it's not the model on which the business was built or now operates. Their chief scientific officer, Karen Miller-Kovach, explained, 'We cannot sustain a business on failure. There's a reason why we have been around fifty years . . . because people come to us time and time again to help them with their chronic condition of weight management.'

One study by Professor Mann for the University of California in Los Angeles analysed thirty-one long-term studies on dieting using a range of popular weight-loss programmes. Her team found that when the researchers checked in on dieters two years after they began their plan the average dieter had already regained 6 of the 12 pounds they had lost. The weight gain continued in the years that followed, and this pattern repeats itself regardless of the diet the individual has been following. Professor Mann's laboratory reviewed sixty years of clinical trials of diets and found people lose an average of 10 per cent of their starting weight on most diets, but within two to five years they have gained back all but about 2 pounds.

This is not to suggest that no one ever successfully loses the weight and keeps it off for several years. The actor Maxine Peake has been open about her weight loss. One of the jobs that brought her to public attention was playing the character of Twinkle in Victoria Wood's sitcom *Dinnerladies*. Maxine told *The Graham Norton Show* that it was Wood who'd prompted her to do something about her weight:

> Victoria said, 'You're fat, you're blonde, you're Northern. You'll get typecast.' She felt it was what she had experienced. I'd been told at drama school, if you don't lay off the chips you'll never play Juliet. I ignored it, I didn't think I wanted to play Juliet, but when someone like Victoria says that to you, you take notice. So I did and lost loads of weight. Anyway, I did Weight Watchers, but unfortunately I did it too quick and had to wear a fat suit for the second series. I'd shifted five stone, but I'm still trying to shake off that image of being big and Northern and being difficult.

Professor Mann says that, based on surveys of those individuals who do stay slim – conducted by Rena Wing at Brown University's Alpert Medical School – the successful ones are far from casual dieters. They tend to make weight loss the complete focus of their lives, weighing themselves and everything they consume every day. They tend to eat the same quantities of the same foods most days, harking back to the original Weight Watchers regime of fish for five days and liver once a week. They also tend to exercise for a minimum of an hour a day, every day.

The dean of Duke University's School of Public Policy, Kelly Brownell, who specializes in obesity, told the *New York Times*, 'They never don't think about their weight.' The weight comes back for all but about 5 per cent of dieters, chiming with Nancy Roberts' assertion, back in 1979, that Weight Watchers, Atkins, Dukan or any other type of diet, faddy or otherwise, has a recidivism rate of 95 per cent.

It's interesting to see the kind of praise and admiration a former fatty engenders in the press when they successfully get rid of a large proportion of their body mass. A great deal of attention has been paid to Tom Watson, the former deputy leader of the Labour Party. Early in 2018 one of his local party members emptied out his own wardrobe and donated to Watson a variety of clothes in considerably smaller sizes so he would have something to fit him for an appearance at Prime Minister's Questions the following week.

At his heaviest Watson weighed 22 stone and in just over a year he lost 7 of them. He explains that for twenty-five years he struggled with his weight, but it was a diagnosis of type 2 diabetes in late 2015 that prompted him to do something radical about the problem. He'd experienced warning signs as his weight and blood pressure increased, but described being told by his doctor that he had the disease – and that his weight was almost certainly the root of his difficulties – as a blow. 'The overwhelming emotion was shame,' he told me. 'I felt frightened and ashamed that I had come to this point. I've only admitted it publicly now, even though I've been in remission for a year, and I've felt quite nervous about discussing it. I think particularly men find it difficult to talk about health.'

After his diagnosis he started taking medication, like so many of the some 3.7 million people in the UK living with type 2 diabetes, but did very little else about it. He believes his attempts to ignore the problem were the result of lack of knowledge, and fear. For a couple of years he was in denial, but then began to read about the illness and realized that if he could get his weight down it would affect his insulin levels and blood pressure. The causes and dangers of type 2 diabetes, and the sense of shame about obesity, which keeps sufferers away from their doctors, is a huge issue to which we'll return in Chapter 8.

Watson found two books helpful. The first was *The Pioppi Diet*, written by cardiologist Dr Aseem Malhotra and Donal O'Neill. It is inspired by the southern Italian village of Pioppi, said to be the healthiest place on the planet, where the inhabitants have a lifespan ten years above average and enjoy a varied diet and a glass of wine every evening. It has echoes of Professor Tim Spector and Dr Michael Mosley, author of *The Fast Diet*, and their keenness for the Mediterranean style of eating. Malhotra puts much of the blame for the rise in heart disease and type 2 diabetes in the UK and the US down to the popularity of the low-fat movement, which began in the 1970s. The basis of his diet is the breaking of the sugar-and-refined-carbohydrate cycle, eating a varied diet (including unrefined fats) when you're hungry and stopping eating when you're full. Susie Orbach again. No snacking in between meals.

The core principles of the plan, and the book says results can be achieved within twenty-one days, are:

1. Go cold turkey on all added sugars for two weeks, cutting out all bread, pasta and rice.
2. No snacking, but eat until you feel full.
3. Make sure you eat 2–4 tablespoons of extra-virgin olive oil every day and a small handful of nuts.
4. As there's no fear of fat, you can eat butter, cheese and full-fat yogurt.
5. Walk for at least thirty minutes a day.
6. Get seven hours of sleep a night.

Watson cut out all refined sugar and the processed foods that often contain hidden sugar. He threw out all his snacks and products such as pasta. He occasionally has brown rice and some pasta when he's out. If he eats bread it's made with almond flour. After three months his diabetes was in remission and he felt much healthier. Now, of course, the trick is trying to keep the weight off.

It's clear that eating in this way becomes a life-long commitment, and Watson is doing far more exercise than a mere half-hour walk a day. As Professor Mann suggests, weight loss has become the focus of his life. He began by taking the stairs rather than lifts and found it wasn't easy at the start. He says he'd forgotten it was thirty-six steps up to his office and the first time he did it he felt he would probably need oxygen at the top. He also began to monitor his daily steps – 10,000 was his target. He began to cycle, and in January 2018 joined a gym and began weight training.

He now does two cardio workouts each week and walks a lot. Being a busy MP and deputy party leader included long hours and travelling, things which can make mindful eating difficult. If he's ever in a position where he can't plan his meals – for example, when he's on a train – he'll order a chicken sandwich and eat only the chicken and maybe a bag of raw nuts. His diet is now adapted to suit him, but sugar is the one thing he's determined he will never eat again. 'My will is very strong on this,' he says. 'It doesn't really challenge me.'

He doesn't count calories and tries to follow a diet of low-glycaemic-index (GI) foods. The index is a number from 0 to 100 assigned to a food, where pure glucose is given the value of 100. Low GI is 55 or less, high is 70 or more. Most veg, fruits, seed, nuts and whole grains are low; most white rice and breakfast cereals would be high. So, Watson will choose berries rather than a banana and has developed a taste for cauliflower rice.

Watson accepts the diet he's created for himself, based on Mediterranean principles, may not work for everyone, but he says one thing he's learned is that 'one-size-fits-all public health advice on nutrition doesn't really work'. He believes it's time GPs are trained to give advice that's tailored to the individual and is keen for food labelling to be improved. He says, 'I hate the fact that people are judged for being overweight when there's a whole load of hidden sugar in processed foods. How does Coca-Cola get away with selling cans containing 35 grams of sugar when the government is telling people an adult should consume no more than 30 grams a day? And this stuff is being sold to kids.'

Another Tom was happy to talk to me about his triumphant weight loss. Tom Kerridge. Tom is the chef who runs the only pub with two Michelin stars – the Hand and Flowers in Marlow, Buckinghamshire. He describes himself as 'a big bloke' and says he rather likes his size. He was always big, even as a child. He's now 6 foot 3 and his weight, by his late thirties, had risen to 30 stone. He had no health concerns, had always been active and worked sixteen- to eighteen-hour days to make a success of his business. He acknowledges he had a serious problem with alcohol – an easy trap to fall into when you run a pub, as it's constantly available and at the end of a hectic day in the kitchen it's the obvious method of winding down. It did, though, occur to him that he was creating problems that would probably hit his health much later in life and he decided to act before those health shocks began.

First he became a teetotaller, giving up alcohol altogether. He had no surgery or gastric band, but created his own low-carbohydrate diet, cutting out all bread, potatoes, pasta and sugars. He eats some fruit, but in moderation. His preferred form of exercise is swimming. He gave it up at one point and began weight-lifting to build muscle, but then went back to it as he lost weight and got down to 19 stone. At forty-six years old, it now fluctuates between 19 and 20.

It has, he says, been incredibly difficult, but also surprisingly easy, which he puts down to an active, aggressive mentality and continually reminding himself that he has to have that kind of positive mind to make such a success of his business. In recent years he's changed from being strictly low-carbohydrate to counting calories. He can now eat whatever he chooses, but counts the exact number of calories in every item of food. The average man needs to eat 2,500 calories a day to maintain his weight, and 2,000 to lose 1 pound each week. The average woman needs 2,000 to maintain and 1,500 to lose. Tom sticks to 2,000. There are, he says, no cheat days. If he wants to eat fish and chips he can, but that would be his full calorie allowance for the day, and even then it would have to be a small portion.

It has to be an obsession in order to keep the weight off, he tells me. He compares it to facing an FA Cup final or a world championship boxing match every single day. Don't close your eyes, he says, or you'll get a left hook. He has to be completely selfish. No matter how much people try to persuade him to eat, drink and be merry at a birthday party, wedding or any other kind of celebration, he cannot be persuaded to deviate from his plan. If he's invited out for a curry with friends he can go, but it's a small portion with very little plain, boiled rice, and only water to drink. 'I have to be confident,' he says. 'I got myself into this, I'll get myself out of it, and it'll mean mental attention to it, all day, every day, for the rest of my life.'

As Kelly Brownell said, 'Successful dieters never don't think about their weight.'

3

The Diet Rollercoaster

Nineteen sixty-eight and I've passed the required number of A levels to begin a joint French and Drama honours degree course at Hull University, the first in my family to go on to higher education, and my parents and grandparents are beside themselves with pride. It had been tough to persuade my mother that studying drama would be a worthwhile idea, as she couldn't imagine what kind of 'sensible' career it might lead to. She'd hoped for a daughter who would teach. She had blocked my ambition to attend drama school with the threat to withdraw all financial support. Reluctantly, she accepted that studying my passion as an academic subject, alongside another, might be OK. There would be funds. I wasn't going to starve!

And so began the trip towards what the Americans call 'freshman 15' and Australia and New Zealand have dubbed 'fresher spread', 'fresher 5' (kilos) or 'first-year fatties'. I had really no excuse for the terrible diet I inflicted upon myself. I knew how to cook nutritious healthy meals, but I quickly fell into a pattern that matched almost exactly what students say about themselves today. In the student magazine *The Tab*, a 2015 survey headed 'Did you get fat during freshers – Pot Noodle anyone?' confirmed that the average fresher will gain

14–28 pounds in their first year, or 1–2 stone. So my own shift from 9½ to 11½ stone is not unusual.

I was hardly aware of it happening. Leaving home at the age of eighteen and having to fend for yourself for the first time introduces a mass of worries and anxieties. I was only too well aware of my family's expectations, given I was the only one to have progressed so far in education. 'How will I manage? Will I make friends? Will I be lonely? Will everybody else be cleverer than me? Can I cope with the work? Will I have enough to live on?' Frankly, feeding yourself well tends to be at the bottom of any list of priorities.

My clearest memories of leaving home are of it being an entirely solitary affair. When my own children left for university, we – their father and I – were there to help. Bags containing clothes, sheets and duvets were loaded into the car along with guitars and Xboxes and books. At their student halls we helped them unpack, checked out the kitchen and made sure there was good food in the fridge for them to get started. We'd already taken great care to ensure they knew basic recipes and methods for putting together a good meal. Eventually we were forced to leave, sobbing, when it became clear we had served our purpose and were merely getting in the way of them beginning their exciting new lives.

It was not like that in my day. I had one suitcase packed with everything I would need for the first term. Mum and Dad were abroad, in Turkey, where Dad was working. Grandma and Grandpa, with whom I'd been living, had no car and neither of them knew how to drive. There was no question of splashing out on a taxi. They saw me to the bus stop, I took the bus into Barnsley, walked around the corner to the railway station and hopped on the train to Leeds. A quick change there for the Hull service and off to a completely strange environment I'd never so much as visited.

In the late sixties it was not common for prospective students to check out beforehand the institutions to which they might apply. School gave advice on which ones they felt would be most suitable in terms of academic requirements and distance from home. They helped to fill out the UCCA form, in it went and you hoped for the best. In my case only four universities offered the course I was desperate to follow. In each case drama – not yet considered serious enough for special degree status – had to be studied as a joint degree and I opted for French and Drama. I didn't want to go to Manchester or Birmingham, Bristol rejected me (I had fun with that when they offered Dame Jenni an honorary degree!) and it was Hull that came up with the goods without even taking the trouble to interview me.

I was pleased to be staying in Yorkshire and impressed by what I'd read about the drama course there. It was relatively young – only three years old – and had a brand-new, state-of-the-art theatre financed by the Gulbenkian Foundation, set up in 1956 in the name of a Portugal-based oil magnate with the aim of funding the arts, philanthropy, science and education. There were rehearsal rooms, and radio and television studios were soon to open. I knew I would enjoy the French – I'd loved learning the language at school – but it was the drama that really thrilled me. I'd studied speech and drama from when I was tiny, had appeared in every school play, and went to the theatre whenever I got the chance. I was full of excitement and enthusiasm.

A number of nervous young people got off the train and looked around anxiously for the coach we'd been promised to take us to our respective student accommodation. Mine was a student house. I was to share a room with a complete stranger, also a fresher. There were two third-year students of theology who would also be resident. They each had their own room. The other double room was occupied by two other first-years, both studying English. There was a well-equipped kitchen and one bathroom and we weren't too far from the shops. It was a good fifteen-minute walk to the campus.

Off we new girls went to the Student Union to find out what was on offer for Freshers' Week. There were clubs to join – I didn't, I've never been a particularly clubbable person, but I did, pretty quickly, find other people who were joining the drama department, hanging about and trying to look trendy and, maybe, a bit dramatic. We seemed to be attracted to each other like iron filings to a magnet.

The parties and dances began and so came my introduction to a drinking culture. Yes, of course I'd been to pubs before. My favourite haunt in Barnsley had been the folk club, held on the upper floor of the Wheatsheaf in the middle of town, but I'd never had anything more than a single vodka and lime that had lasted me the whole evening and which wouldn't smell on my breath when I got home, giving me away to my mother. Anyway, my friend Linda and I couldn't have afforded anything more.

Suddenly, we all had money in our pockets as the student maintenance grant had come through in good time, and the Union bar was notoriously cheap. It was the meeting place for everyone who was out to have a good time. It was a few drinks before a dance or a party and, although I was never fond of beer, I went along with everybody else. Maybe one vodka to start, or a glass of wine, then a couple of half-pints. They wouldn't serve full pints to women, which was infuriating and I doubt any landlord/lady would dare to impose such a rule today, but it might have been a blessing in disguise for my waistline, because even with that relatively small amount of alcohol I was racking up my calorie count.

The 2015 article in *The Tab* described how Freshers' Week flashes by in a blur of vodka, kebabs, sex and culinary disasters: 'Suddenly there is no one pushing you to eat your five a day or stocking the fridge with healthy food and, with only a crash course in the basics from Mum or Dad under your belt, a lot of us are pretty clueless when it comes to the kitchen. Takeaways and microwave meals become the norm.'

Of course we didn't have a microwave in 1968, nor was there something I also learned from *The Tab* is now available for students: free junk food. 'It would be silly not to make the most of the free cheeseburger you can get with your student card when you buy a meal at Maccies. The lack of regularity in meals and late-night snacking are among the biggest contributors to weight gain.' We had the Wimpy Bar, the chippy, the canteen and the toaster in the house. And that turned out to be plenty.

An evening out meant something stodgy with chips in the canteen, going out drinking, a quick fish and chips on the way home and then, because students don't go to sleep when the pubs shut, having mates back to the house – Bob Dylan or Joan Baez on the record player, maybe a bottle of wine or beer to share and enough buttered toast to feed an army. Eating out was a rare event but would mean a trip to the local Chinese restaurant. One portion of sweet and sour pork shared between two and a plate of boiled rice each. I don't honestly remember doing any cooking at all.

I thought lots of exercise would keep me fit and slim. Our first weekend in the drama department was a punishing forty-eight hours of brutal exercises controlled by the dance teacher to prepare us for the fact that we would soon be expected to do a performance of Stravinsky's *Rite of Spring*. The drama course would challenge us academically and physically and, with no means of transport other than Shanks' pony, there'd be lots of walking. I had no doubt I'd be fine.

It's funny how you seem not to really notice yourself putting on weight. You see yourself in the mirror every day, but, of course, it just creeps up on you. You notice weight gain in friends and family, but not so much in yourself. Maybe you genuinely don't notice it or maybe it's just that you kid yourself that the old familiar face hasn't changed at all because you really don't want to acknowledge it.

My style of dressing was to copy the Bohemian fashion of the French actor and singer Juliette Gréco – black pants, black baggy sweater, long black (well, nearly) hair and pronounced black eyeliner. I looked in the mirror and saw nothing concealed under my chosen uniform to worry about. It was when my parents came home for the Easter holidays, two-thirds of the way through that first year, that all hell broke loose.

They had decided to drive back to the UK from Istanbul, where Dad had been working. It was a journey of 1,677 miles, taking in Eastern Europe from Bulgaria, through Serbia, Hungary, Austria and Germany, then the North Sea Ferry from Rotterdam to Hull. I would be waiting for them at the ferry terminal.

I got up early, had some breakfast, tidied myself up as best I could, took the bus to the right place and arrived in good time. I stood waiting as car after car disembarked, peering through endless windscreens to see if I could spot my mother and father. I hadn't thought to ask what type of car they'd be driving. They'd hired their transport and picked it up in Turkey, so it wasn't a vehicle with which I was familiar. Eventually they appeared and drove straight past me. I ran after them. Mercifully they were going very slowly, obviously keeping an eye out for their beloved daughter. I shouted and waved frantically. Finally my father spotted me in his rear-view mirror. He stopped the car. He jumped out. He hugged me. My mother didn't. She remained in the car, stony-faced.

'Come on, love,' said my dad. 'Jump in. We can't wait to see where you're living and find out everything about what you're up to.'

My heart had sunk to my boots. Why had Mum not jumped out to greet me? I hadn't seen her for months. Why did she look so furious? No one knew how to wear their heart on their sleeve like my mother. There was no way she was going to hide her displeasure, but I had really no idea what I'd done to upset her to this extent.

I climbed into the back seat behind her. She said nothing. Dad began to pull away. She turned around and looked at me with utter disdain. 'What the hell has happened to you?' she asked. I was mystified. Was it the long hair? Was it the eye make-up? Were the clothes I wore not smart or elegant enough for her? No. She spat out the words. 'You look absolutely awful. You look like a baby elephant.'

Dad did his best to smooth things over. 'Oh, come on, Win, she looks fine. We've so been looking forward to seeing her. What's the matter with you? She's your daughter. Please don't be horrible.'

'She doesn't look like any daughter of mine,' Mum moaned.

'Look at her, Alvin. She looks like the side of a house. For goodness' sake, she's fat!'

I looked down at myself. My God, she was right. Why hadn't it occurred to me to diet before she got home?

We drove to the student house. A cursory glance around. Dad wanted to see the campus. We walked there. My mother showed no interest whatsoever in anything I showed them and simply moved from stunned silence to a constant, furious tirade, telling me how appalled she was that I had let myself go so badly. Did I want to end up looking like Grandma and being as round as I was tall?

After a couple of hours of this, none of us could take any more. Dad asked me if I wanted to come home with them for the weekend. I said no, I was busy. My mother looked relieved that she wouldn't have to look at me any more. They drove away. I spent the afternoon in my room in shocked silence, unable to bring myself to do anything but lie there, sobbing.

I can't say I felt heartbroken at being fat shamed by my own mother. The term didn't exist in the late sixties but, with hindsight, that's exactly what had happened. My mother, the woman who was supposed to love me unconditionally and care enough to wonder what might have been making me so unhappy or unsure of myself that I had eaten myself to that size, had nothing to offer but disappointment and shame. She was truly ashamed of me and my heart was breaking. It's an object lesson in how not to treat your own child and a weight problem. I've never forgotten it and it didn't stop there. That evening I had a phone call from her, still fuming.

'I just thought I'd let you know what trouble you've caused.' She was so angry she could hardly get the words out. 'We got as far as Selby and Dad was so upset about you and the state you're in he ran into the back of another car. Luckily no one was injured, but I hope you're pleased with yourself for causing so much upset.'

She hung up.

I wasn't sure I was the one who'd caused all the upset. I hadn't spoken to anyone in a completely vile and hurtful way. She had. I didn't think I would ever forgive her for her over-reaction when we had all been so excited about seeing each other again. I'm not really sure I ever did. But I made a decision. When I saw them again at the end of the summer term I would no longer be fat.

I truly hadn't worried about my weight gain until my mother made so much of it. Maybe we can only be prompted into making an effort to change when someone else points it out and makes us feel ashamed, although the evidence suggests that fat shaming can have precisely the opposite effect and make us sink into more misery and comfort eating. In my case, I wasn't going to risk another similar encounter with my mother and her criticisms. I made up my mind that I was going to do something about it. I did.

My first stop was the university medical centre. I saw a young GP, told him everything that had happened with my mother, and found him to be warm and sympathetic. He told me to pop on to the weight scales. It was quite a shock. I weighed 11½ stone.

'You're right,' he said. 'That's too much for someone of your height and build, but I can do something to help you with it. I'll give you a prescription for some pills that will help you diet. You'll soon be fine again.'

I'm sure I knew instinctively what I needed to do to lose weight. We all know instinctively what we need to do to lose weight – especially if it's only a little that needs to be lost. Eat less and move more is often heralded as the simple solution, although we now know it doesn't always work and new scientific research tells us why. More of the complications of weight loss and dieting later.

I knew, though, that I'd been raised by wonderful cooks who understood the importance of fruit, vegetables and preparing good-quality fresh food, and a return to that life, using my own culinary skills, would have been the best option. But I wanted to do things quickly. There was no time for a long-haul programme of sensible eating and exercise. I was a mess, at least in my mother's eyes, and I had no intention of enduring another of her angry reproaches.

There are lots of reasons for wanting to lose weight. As I grew older, like so many of us, I wanted to be able to move more easily and to no longer feel that my weight was a health risk that might shorten my life. Some of us just live by the Kate Moss mantra that 'nothing tastes as good as skinny feels', but I suspect that most of us simply want to match up to the assumption that slim is the way we should all be and will devote ourselves to trying to fit the stereotype.

Of course I wanted to look gorgeous and have boys fancy me, but curiously, there hadn't been any problems in that department, despite my weight gain. No, for me, it was that aching desire to make my mother proud. She had, to be honest, made me realize that I was not really happy to be a lumbering late teenager.

I picked up the pills from the chemist, took them as instructed, found very quickly that I had hardly any appetite at all and looked through a selection of women's magazines to see what diets were on trend.

I came across one that seemed really simple and cheap. You had to drink plenty of tea, coffee and water – no booze, no milk and definitely no sugar – and at each mealtime you were allowed to eat one boiled egg and a chopped tomato. Easy peasy. I would turn myself into Twiggy. That'd show that mother of mine!

There were a good few crazy diets in the 1960s. Nineteen sixty itself had seen the introduction of the cabbage soup diet. It had to be eaten three or four times a day. It was disgusting and was widely reported to cause dizziness and fatigue. You lost weight, as the soup was mostly water, but that meant such a regime couldn't be sustained. In 1962, Helen Gurley Brown, later the editor of *Cosmopolitan*, recommended a diet in her book *Sex and the Single Girl*. Breakfast was an egg in any style, but with no butter, and one glass of white wine. The same for lunch. Dinner was a steak and another glass of white wine. She said it would make you sexy, exuberant and full of *joie de vivre*. I doubt it! Pretty drunk for most of the day, I suspect.

The Drinking Man's Diet by Robert Cameron was published in the mid-sixties and sold more than 2 million copies in only two years. It recommended eating 'manly, protein-rich foods such as steak and lobster, accompanied by as much alcohol as you choose'. It was the first popular low-carb diet and was definitely designed to please the hard-drinking male executive who had already developed a paunch. It was followed in 1967 by *The Stillman Diet* by Dr Irwin Maxwell Stillman, which was published years before the Atkins diet and similarly allowed lean cuts of meat and low-fat dairy. It became very popular when Karen Carpenter used it to lose weight. As we know, unfortunately she died not long after, having developed anorexia.

There were, at times, warnings about the dangers of following fads. It was in 1968 that diet pills became popular, although *Life* magazine issued a warning. On 26 January 1968 its front cover featured a silhouette of a rotund woman with pills scattered throughout her head and body. The headline read 'The dangerous diet pills – how millions of women are risking their health with fat doctors.' I didn't bother to read it. I trusted the university's own medical centre. Surely someone trained to take care of students wouldn't be dishing out anything that would be risky.

It's curious that so many of us have complete faith in medicine and science, but the weight-loss industry has seen its fair share of snake-oil salesmen who've convinced us that their diet plan, their medication, or their research paper on foods and how to cook them will be the Holy Grail to keeping us slim. Anyone who reads the newspapers or magazines is only too aware of the extent to which studies can contradict each other and how information keeps changing. I hope I've learned, after that awful first experience, to choose my scientists and their advice very carefully. There's a whole chapter on the most recent science later in the book and I've only included information from people in whom I've put my trust.

I had a repeat prescription for the diet pills so I didn't have to go back to the surgery to have my progress checked. The weight simply fell off and, because I was still following the drama department's super-active physical training programme, I didn't end up with flabby bits from where the excess fat had disappeared. I felt great. I was full of energy, I got on with my work and people kept telling me how incredibly good I looked. Ah yes, the power of other people's approval!

And then, after a couple of months, coming up to the end-of-first-year exams, they stopped telling me I looked good. Nobody mentioned the way I looked at all. Nobody suggested I join them in the canteen or at the bar. They knew I would refuse and say I had to get back to my desk to get on with some work. My housemates made no reference to the oddly limited amount of food I kept in the fridge. I became a difficult person with whom to have a conversation and the wonderfully high marks I'd had for my essays at the beginning of the year began to slip.

I was totally unaware of how bizarre my behaviour must have seemed to other people, and I can only assume it was the power of the diet pills that made me oblivious to my poor performance and up-and-down emotions. All I could think about was how slim I was getting.

My tutor, John Harris, who was responsible for my pastoral care, eventually stepped in. He called me into his room. I thought he'd have something funny and encouraging to say about how my figure was improving. He'd joked with our seminar group one day about how difficult he'd found it to eat a decent diet at Oxford. He'd survived for a whole year on Guinness, and baked beans on toast. It hadn't done him any harm, he'd told us.

He had not called me in to pay me compliments. 'Jenni,' he said, with a truly worried tone in his voice, 'what's going on with you? You're a different person from the one who came to me at the beginning of the academic year. You've become painfully thin, I've noticed you often seem to be upset and a bit tearful, and your work, which was of such a high quality, has really deteriorated. What drugs are you on?'

I was horrified. There wasn't a huge drug problem at the

university, although a cannabis joint would occasionally appear at parties and I knew some of my more adventurous colleagues had had a go with LSD. They'd followed the advice, delivered in 1967 by the hero of the hippy counter-culture Timothy Leary, to 'turn on, tune in and drop out'. I certainly wasn't one of the 'druggies'. I hadn't even had a puff on a joint. I knew it gave you the munchies and an uncontrollable long-ing for sweets and chocolate. That would have entirely defeated my slimming plan. I would have been far too scared to take psychedelic substances such as LSD or mescaline, Aldous Huxley's choice of substance for opening 'the doors of percep-tion'. I remember one of my friends telling me he'd had the most terrifying trip, which went on for almost twenty-four hours. He'd stood in front of the mirror and almost frightened himself to death watching himself age and become an old, old man.

'No,' I said most emphatically to John. 'I don't take drugs. Well, apart from the pills the doctor at the health centre pre-scribed to help me lose weight.'

'Show me,' he said. I had them in my handbag. I showed him.

'Good God, Jenni!' He was horrified. 'Those are bloody Black Bombers. Stop taking them this minute.'

I had to ask him to explain what a Black Bomber was. I had no idea. He told me they were very powerful amphetamines and he could now see exactly why I was in such a state. He whisked me off to the health centre, made a vociferous com-plaint, and got me to see an older and wiser doctor who was shocked to find I weighed just under 7 stone. No one used the word 'anorexia', but they did say I needed to be admitted to the health centre for a week or two to be slowly brought back to a normal eating pattern. They then wanted me to go home and be cared for by my mother. I didn't want her to know what a mess I was in and I insisted I would be capable of sitting the end-of-term exams after a short stay in the health centre. I was adamant.

Learning how to eat again was not an easy task and the withdrawal symptoms from the ghastly amphetamines were horrific. I lay in the bed in the health centre weeping and shivering with fear. Every bone in my body ached and at night, in the dark, I was terrified of being alone and begged to be given something to make me feel better, to get rid of the headaches and the pain that wracked me through and through. I was refused all medication. I think their policy was what's known as going cold turkey.

In the mornings I was given coffee with milk and sugar. I've always hated sugar in hot drinks, but they seemed to think stuffing me with calories was probably the only way to build me up again. They brought porridge with honey, and toast and marmalade. By the end of the two weeks I could just about manage a couple of spoonfuls of the porridge, but left the toast untouched. Lunch was tomato or vegetable soup, and tea was a couple of sandwiches and a cake. I didn't eat the cake and barely managed half a sandwich. In the early evening they would bring me dinners of meat, potatoes and two veg, which was really difficult to manage, although I did begin to regain a sense of smell and taste, which had all but deserted me towards the end of my diet.

There's no doubt the whole experience was deeply shocking. I knew I was a competent, often courageous and intelligent young woman. How had I allowed myself to 'let myself go', to use my mother's terminology, and then fall into the idea that a doctor could be trusted entirely to do his best for me? Why had I not questioned the impact amphetamines can have? Why had I not read the information in the package that might have warned of side effects? Why, with my knowledge of drugs and the dangers they can present, was I not aware of the effect they were having on my mental, as well as my physical, health?

I can only think it was an act of desperation, because I was so hurt by my mother's behaviour. It gave me a good lesson in how not to damage your child's confidence – a lesson we perhaps all need to learn. Kind and gentle guidance, I think, is so much more effective than making demands with anger. It was also a lesson in who to trust. If I hadn't listened to my tutor and taken his advice, I doubt I would ever have recovered from the dreadful state I was in. Sometimes you just have to accept that there are people who have your best interests at heart and follow their lead.

Towards the end of the second week I reiterated my intention to discharge myself and go ahead with my plan to complete the end-of-year exams. I had put on a couple of pounds and didn't feel quite as weak as I had when they'd admitted me. I was still weepy and shaky, but mental-health questions were rarely raised in the late sixties. It was a question of 'pull yourself together', and get up and get on with things.

Thankfully we have become much more aware of how fragile mental health can be, although it's still not the priority in the NHS it perhaps should be. I was just told to make sure to eat properly and to stay away from any drugs. As I walked out of the little ward I made a vow to myself. I would cook and eat sensibly, I would take care with alcohol, never take drugs and never allow a boiled egg and a tomato to share space on the same plate again. I would also never go on another trendy fad diet. I stuck to those resolutions for a good few years and, even now, I can eat a boiled egg and a tomato, but never together. The mere thought makes me want to be sick.

I finished the exams and did OK. My tutor, John, was very supportive and went through my papers when the results came out. I'd managed to make the equivalent of a 2:2 even in the pathetic state I'd been in. He reassured me I would definitely be 2:1 or even first material if I took good care of myself and worked hard. He made one other demand of me. To spend the summer holidays in my mother's care at home.

I was nineteen years old, determined to assert my independence, and the last thing on earth I wanted to do was place myself under my mother's supervision for the long vacation. I had done what she demanded and made myself thin, but I had no doubt that our first encounter would be fraught with unease on both our parts. I almost talked myself out of going home, but the power of that word, 'home', is strong. It means love, comfort and care, and you long for it even though deep in your heart you know it will come with a lot of discomfort and pain. Nevertheless, it made sense from the perspective of my health. There would be good food and memories of happy times at the dining table before I created my own eating disaster area.

Before I could go away on the holiday I had planned with a friend came the moment of truth – turning up at my mother's house and having her see how very slender I was. 'Oh, Jen,' she said. 'My poor love. What have you done to yourself? You are painfully thin.' Couldn't she just have said, 'Hello, my love, it's so good to see you', without any reference to my size? Of course she couldn't. By now I had managed to put on a good half-stone and was weighing in at around 7½ stone. I decided to go on the offensive, in the hope that she'd realize how much damage she'd done. I told her in great detail exactly what I'd done to myself and why.

I explained how very upset I'd been by her response to my weight gain when we'd met in Hull, and that it had made me determined to sort myself out and make myself slim again. I told her about the doctor who'd given me the amphetamines, the response of my tutor, the fact that I'd been admitted to the university's health centre and that I'd insisted on confidentiality. My parents were not to be informed, I had told the medical staff. I had wanted, I told my mother, to be responsible for myself and I would continue to do so. I was now an adult and no longer 'her project'.

She seemed to be a little upset at the business with the drugs and said how she hoped the doctor who'd prescribed them would be struck off. She refused, though, to accept that my misery had had anything to do with her flood of insults about my weight and the phone call in which she'd blamed me for Dad's distress and the little shunt they'd had in the car at Selby. It was my fault for 'having let myself go' and now, 'typically', I had gone too far in the other direction. It was not going to be an easy summer as we went through her determined efforts to 'fatten you up a bit, but not too much'.

I doubt very much that I'm alone in carrying my mother's words with me and feeling every verbal slap in the face no matter how old I get. Nor can I entirely absolve myself of guilt as a mother. One day, I'm sure, my boys will come back at me with the painful words they hold in their hearts. We should all be so much more aware of the hurt we can engender for a lifetime.

The regime she insisted upon was 'three good meals a day'. Bacon and egg (no tomatoes or toast) for breakfast, ham and salad for lunch with one slice of bread and margarine, then at tea time there was a cup of tea and a small slice of home-made chocolate cake or a buttered scone, and for dinner there was meat or fish with vegetables, or a shepherd's pie or chicken casserole. It was, on the whole, a delicious and carefully balanced diet and I managed to gain another stone. It wasn't easy to get back into a pattern of eating according to her rules, but I knew I had made myself ill and much too thin. If getting my strength back meant going along with every 'come on, eat up, it's good for you', I was determined to go along with her.

I'd made an arrangement with a good friend to take his car up the east coast for a couple of weeks in August. We'd visit Amble for the crabs and fresh fish, Alnwick for the castle, Craster for the kippers, and finish up at Berwick-upon-Tweed. Then we'd travel back to Yorkshire inland, through the hills of the Northumberland National Park, the North Pennines and the Yorkshire Dales.

The best part of the whole holiday was relaxing on the beautiful beach at Bamburgh with the castle rising above us and having a dip in the freezing-cold North Sea. It was a gloriously sunny August bank holiday and we were the only people on the beach. I had no fear of being seen in a swimsuit now I considered myself neither too thin nor too fat, and began to feel I could put the lessons learned from the appallingly bad university diet to good use. I ate whatever I fancied on the trip, but never to excess.

It was such a significant place for me, as a scene from my favourite film of all time was shot there: the meeting between Thomas à Becket and Henry II, played in the movie *Becket* by Richard Burton and Peter O'Toole. Historically the two had met to try to resolve their differences on a beach in Normandy. In the film, Bamburgh was used as the location and I loved the moment in which my two most admired actors of the time galloped towards each other along the whole length of the long golden sands of Northumberland. I still remember lying there in the sun, picturing the two lovely men galloping right past me. I had adored the film, and the place, the memories and a new-found confidence in my appearance made me the happiest I'd felt in a long time.

Returning to university in September, I was at a very happy weight. For several years I ranged between 9 and 9½ stone, feeding myself with great care, drinking in moderation and getting plenty of exercise. I didn't learn to drive until I was twenty-three, so I did lots of walking, carried on riding whenever I could and took up yoga too. I knew what to do to keep the weight off, and I did my best.

That period of my life unquestionably did untold damage to my relationship with my mother. She became obsessed with my size and the way I looked, and was never able to resist making a comment, which would rarely be complimentary. The moment I arrived at her house it would be, 'Oh Lord, you've got fat again,' or, as my weight frequently went up and down as I got older and stepped on to the dieting rollercoaster, it would be, 'Oh, you've lost weight. A bit too much, if you want my opinion.'

She was very impressed and proud as my career advanced. She cut out every article about me, but would always phone to say whether she thought the photo had flattered me or not. 'Bit thin in the *Mail*' or 'What was that *Telegraph* photographer thinking? Your double chin looked awful.' When I began to work on national television as a presenter of *Newsnight*, she almost drove me crazy with her comments about my appearance.

I like to think she was trying to express her love for me, that she cared enough about me to want me always to look my best. I'm not convinced. In retrospect, I believe there were elements of jealousy. I was engaged in interesting work, which she had been bright enough to do but never had the opportunity. I doubt it ever occurred to her that the constant criticism hurt me and dashed my confidence on an almost daily basis.

Radio was such a relief. She could hear me, but she couldn't see me. I love working on the radio, but I suspect my determination to make it the main part of my career and largely leave television behind was informed by the response to my appearance being constantly highlighted by my mother. I could hide behind the microphone. I remember being adamant when it was suggested that we should have a camera in the *Woman's Hour* studio when live streaming became a thing. 'No! Radio has no pictures. The listeners make up their own.' I still feel the same way and always dread having publicity photos taken.

Mum's behaviour continued to the very end of her life. In my late forties and early fifties she suffered from Parkinson's. I had a job, a husband and teenage children to care for. I tried to see her nearly every weekend to help my father care for her, but no matter how hard I tried to help her deal with her condition she never welcomed me without an 'Oh, good grief, Jen, you're back to being a baby elephant again. For goodness' sake, do something about it.' Virtually the last words she said to me just before she died at the end of 2005, when I was fifty-five, were: 'You are so selfish. You only think about yourself and the bloomin' BBC. And isn't it time you went on a diet?'

4

Comfort and Eating

It was in my forties that my problems with weight gain began to be serious once more. Middle-age spread is no fantasy. It might be a beer belly, a spare tyre or a muffin top – horrible names – but it's not uncommon, as in our thirties and forties the levels of hormones that maintain muscle mass begin to fall off. We also tend to become less active, so our muscles suffer from lack of use. Then there's the extra consumption of food. Professor Tim Gill at the Boden Institute of Obesity, Nutrition, Exercise and Eating Disorders at the University of Sydney says that as we age, we tend to eat as a distraction or as a pastime rather than because we're hungry. It's a recipe for weight gain without regular weight-bearing exercises – push-ups, Pilates, weight-lifting and taking the stairs. Never a favoured pastime for me.

After that dreadful time at university and the experience of losing so much weight on an absolutely ridiculous diet with insane medical advice, I'd done my best to keep to a weight with which I felt comfortable. I kept my vow never to submit myself to another fierce dieting regime. I would simply be sensible. I would avoid junk food, eat on the whole whatever I fancied, but keep the portions to a reasonably moderate size. Drinking would be allowed, but again, moderation would be the watchword.

I had, by now, learned to drive a car, but still walked a lot and frequently used public transport. Through my twenties and thirties I continued to horse ride as often as I could, which kept my core strong and my thighs trim, and yoga was the one regular form of exercise – apart from horses – that I found enjoyable. I was extremely supple and fit, and able to sleep well and relax. I managed to keep my weight steady between 9½ and 10½ stone, which is perfectly acceptable for a woman of 5 feet 7 inches. My BMI was 23, and the 'healthy' weight range for someone of my age and height was 8 stone 6 pounds to 11 stone 5 pounds. I was fine. But I never stopped thinking about it.

During my thirties I had two children. Ed was born when I was thirty-three and Charlie when I was thirty-seven. I didn't put on an excessive amount of weight during the two pregnancies, although inevitably there was some expansion, but I kept on doing the yoga and the riding. My deliveries were spectacularly easy and relatively short; Ed in hospital and Charlie at home. I've always assumed it was thanks to being blessed with childbearing hips, but it was mostly because I never gave up on the regular yoga.

After both pregnancies the slight weight gain disappeared relatively quickly. In the eighties there was none of the pressure that new mothers face today to get their pre-baby body back virtually overnight. I don't recall any of the constant pressure we see in the papers these days, caused by the photos of anyone from the Duchess of Cambridge to Amal Clooney or Victoria Beckham looking perfectly lithe and slender only weeks after they've emerged from the delivery room.

It's all too common in this era of what the psychotherapist Susie Orbach describes as a 'body-hating society' for new mothers to long to look as if they've never had a baby. I felt no obligation to 'get my body back'. There was no social media, with celebrities and influencers posting selfies in which they were carefully dressed, perfectly posed, made up to the nines and beautifully lit, to make me feel utterly inadequate. If only the girls, young women and, increasingly, young men who now look at such pictures dozens of times a day were more aware of the hard work and photographic technology required to make those Instagrammers look so 'perfect'.

I'm sure most of them know about photoshopping, where images are manipulated way beyond the reality, but still they want to achieve 'the look'. I would love it if they would simply accept that there are lots of different types of bodies and sizes. As long as they're not dangerously overweight and unfit they should learn to be happy with what and who they are. Size zero should not be the ambition of any healthy young woman or man. Happily, the fad for skinny seems to be diminishing somewhat as strong and healthy look to begin to find their place again.

I was, though, still only in my thirties and wanted to regain some of what had been a far from perfect but decent figure. After all, two months after Ed's birth, I went back to appearing regularly on television and had a mother who kept a beady eye on me constantly. Things were easier after Charlie's birth because by then I had moved from *Newsnight* to the *Today* programme on BBC Radio 4 and then, when he was a few months old, to *Woman's Hour*. Radio, as I said, tends to relieve some of the anxiety about the way you look.

Breastfeeding is, I'm convinced, the best way to begin to get back to your usual size and I was lucky enough to be able to feed both my boys. I could feel, in both cases, the little bit of excess just falling away. It didn't help with tightening up the muscles and the slightly saggy skin, though, so, for the first time in my life, I added gym work to the yoga classes and the horse riding. I dutifully went there twice a week, slogging away on the exercise bike, the treadmill, the cross trainer, and would then go downstairs for half an hour's swim. I hated every minute. It hadn't been my thing at school to take off all my clothes in a changing room with a whole lot of other girls and then have my lack of ability in the fitness game observed by them. And it wasn't my thing in my thirties. Everybody seemed slimmer, fitter and younger than me. I kept it up for a year and then packed it in. I've never been back, except to the pool and the yoga or Pilates classes.

Going to the gym seems to have become something of an obligation in the new world that appears to have gone fitness-crazy. There's a gym on every corner in the cities, big companies offer a workout room in the workplace, you'll find one in fancy new blocks of flats, and 'at the gym' has become a status on WhatsApp. But there's evidence that a vast number of us – primarily women – suffer from what's been dubbed 'gymtimidation'.

Cosmopolitan magazine conducted a survey in December 2012 and found almost half of the women polled were put off going into the gym's weights section because of 'the type of people in them' and 14 per cent said they were intimidated by the thought of men judging them. Similarly, Sport England, launching its 'This Girl Can' campaign, found that of the 9.4 million women aged fourteen to forty in the UK, 75 per cent would like to be more active, but they didn't exercise for fear of being judged. For me, the only solution has been yoga and Pilates. It's important to find an exercise you enjoy – dancing is becoming popular – and preferably one where there aren't too many men staring at you in your Lycra.

Taking care of small children can be an easy way to keep fit and burn off energy. My two boys and our dogs needed lots of fresh air and long walks and, as they were both big, strong babies, just carrying them around was the equivalent of weight-lifting.

Susie Orbach, in *Fat Is a Feminist Issue*, points to the difficulties faced by a lot of young mothers who don't go out to work, stay at home with their children and, like the housewives I lived with – my mother and grandmother – devote themselves to creating wonderful food for their families, gaining pleasure themselves from putting a delicious meal on the table, but often finding they're in the kitchen after everything's been cleared away, hoovering up whatever the kids have wasted.

I didn't have that problem. I was the family breadwinner and my husband, David, always joked that he was the one who made the bread, literally. To be honest, we tended to share responsibility for the shopping and cooking, and we were both extremely careful about what we fed the children and, consequently, ourselves. Of course, there was the inevitable and ever-popular spaghetti bolognese and chilli con carne, which are quick but never on a slimmer's menu, but there was also always plenty of good meat, fish, vegetables and salad, and we tried to keep sugar down to a minimum.

We ate butter not margarine and cooked with olive oil, which we also used for salad dressings. When the fashion for children's birthday parties at McDonald's began, we didn't make a fuss, and never demanded that the boys should avoid any cakes or pastries they might be offered at someone else's house. Grandma's chocolates and sweets were always gratefully received, but we made sure that junk food and sugary sweets and drinks were only a very occasional thing.

It's a way of feeding a family that has received more and more publicity in recent years, and it's fine to expect parents to follow such guidance if they've been taught about what's a good diet and they've learned to prepare it. How did we let domestic science, as it was known in my day, die as a subject in schools – for both girls and boys? Then there's the cost question. It's hard for lots of families to afford food at all, let alone to fork out for the very best.

In my house, if there were sweets or chocolate they were just there, never sold to the kids as 'a treat if you eat your dinner'. That's a dangerous game to play. And we never had any trouble with leftovers. They both had healthy appetites, but if they did leave food on the plate because they were full or simply weren't hungry there was never any pressure to 'eat up'. I didn't want my children to have the unhealthy relationship with processed food that I had developed in my teenage years.

They've both grown up to be wonderful cooks with a great respect for fresh and varied ingredients. I like to think of the way we brought them up as our gift to the women in their adult lives. What could be better than raising a son who understands instinctively the importance of feeding the microbiome and comes to visit prepared to cook a fabulously healthy meal with some good, fresh cheese to finish and a jar of home-made, fermented sauerkraut as a gift? (Try it, it's surprisingly good.)

So, how did it all start to go so wrong for me? Perhaps there's a moment for everyone who sets out on the road to obesity where things begin to get out of control, and it's probably triggered by some big change in one's life. I was forty-one in 1991 when *Woman's Hour*, which I'd presented for four days a week since 1987, moved from the slot it had occupied since its inception in 1946 – two o'clock in the afternoon – to the morning. It was not a popular move, made by the then controller of Radio 4, Michael Green. He had noticed that there had been a bit of a drop in audience figures in the mid-morning and, rightly as it turned out, thought a popular magazine would solve the problem.

There was talk of renaming the programme and changing its focus, but that suggestion generated a lot of anger. Michael ignored the complaints that argued women wouldn't be able to listen in the morning because they would be busy doing noisy jobs such as washing or hoovering, but he did listen to concerns that we should lose the title *Woman's Hour*. Questions about the proposed change of name and focus were tabled in the House of Commons and the then speaker, Betty Boothroyd, got in touch to ask us what she could do to help.

It was a marketing consultant who saved the day. She advised that *Woman's Hour* was a loved and trusted brand, which she compared to Marks & Spencer or Jammy Dodgers. It's OK, she said, to change a brand's packaging or even move a few doors down the street, but you don't change its name. So, we lost on the time change, but kept the title and subject matter.

I firmly believe that time change first influenced my weight problems. Night shifts and very early starts have been shown to increase the risk of obesity. Sleeping during the day disrupts the body's metabolism, causing the worker to use less energy than is normal during the course of a full day and a full night's sleep. Sleeping in the afternoon means between 12 and

16 per cent fewer calories are burned than when sleeping at night.

Dr Kenneth Wright, director of the Sleep and Chronobiology Laboratory at the University of Colorado, says lower energy use may accentuate the poor diet and lack of exercise that is often seen in these workers. He pointed out that his research into the impact of sleep and circadian disruption on the human microbiome had found that 'as little as 50 kcal excess calorie storage per day can increase weight over time and, if increased exhaustion and fatigue levels associated with shift work result in reduced physical activity levels, this would promote weight gain'.

I wasn't working all night, but I had to get up at five every morning. A quick cup of coffee before driving to the studio and a breakfast of plenty of coffee and buttered toast from the canteen, or maybe a couple of croissants and a latte picked up on the way in. The whole morning, from seven o'clock, was spent sitting at a desk in front of a computer. First read the papers, then highly pressured preparation for the programme. Write the script, prepare for the interviews, into the studio – at first at ten thirty, then it changed to ten, which is where it's remained. The broadcast lasts an hour and can also be highly stressful as it's live. After I've said goodbye to the audience there's a meeting to review what's gone out on that morning and then we prepare for the following day.

By lunchtime I would be starving. Sometimes we'd pop up to the canteen for chips with everything. More often the editor and I would go to one of the cheap local restaurants, most frequently for Greek or Turkish food, meaning hummus, pitta bread, fried calamari, chips with a kebab and baklava for pudding, all washed down with a nice bottle of white wine. I don't remember the 'nip out for a sandwich and eat at the desk' culture that seems to dominate eating habits in the twenty-first century.

Snacking, the proliferation of the latte and 'bring in a cake as a treat for your colleagues' can all be lovely trends, but when so many of us sit down for most of the day it can't be doing us any good at all. In those early days of mid-morning *Woman's Hour*, I would go back to the office after lunch for a conversation with the producer of the following day's programme, pick up any books that needed to be read and then be home around three o'clock. Just in time to pick up the kids from school.

Their dad would give them tea whilst I would collapse in a heap in the bed for an hour's sleep. The evening would be spent bathing and putting the children to bed, reading them stories, eating with the old man – he cooked – and bed around eleven. Quite often I had to go to the theatre to see a play we'd be discussing on the programme. I was exhausted and creating a recipe for disaster.

Friday was a day off, but I often found myself sitting at the computer at home, writing articles for a newspaper or putting a book together. I did no exercise apart from the walk to and from the children's school, which was just down the road, riding with the family at Wimbledon Village Stables at the weekend and walking our dogs on Wimbledon Common. Even the yoga, which I'd practised at home almost every day for years, fell by the wayside.

I was forty-three and still presenting *Woman's Hour* four days a week when, in 1993, we decided to leave London. David is a Cheshire man, educated at a solid Northern grammar school, and I had had a rigidly thorough education at Barnsley Girls' High School. We wanted something similar for our boys.

I remembered Brian Redhead, with whom I'd worked for a short time as a presenter of Radio 4's *Today*, raving about a small town called Macclesfield. It was on the edge of the beautiful Peak District and had an excellent train service to London and Manchester – where Ed was to start school. We sold our house in South London and moved to the hills just outside Macclesfield in good time for Ed to begin his first term. I, of course, would become very familiar with the West Coast trains – up and down every week.

There'd been a slight panic in the weeks before we moved out of the London house. There'd been so much to think about that the last thing on my mind was where I would live when I had to be in the capital for work. Then a friend, Kate, who's been my broadcast agent for years, rang to say her brother was leaving a rented flat in Camden Town, for which he'd paid a very reasonable rent. She advised me to write to the landlord. It was a basement in Gloucester Crescent and was really beyond what you might call Bohemian.

There was a sitting room; a bedroom; a tiny bathroom with no bath, just a shower; and a kitchen, which was falling apart. Its main selling point was a huge 100-foot garden that needed some attention. It would be something to occupy me and somewhere to get fresh air in the summer. The lovely landlord agreed to a new ceiling being put up in the sitting room and a total renovation of the kitchen. I would provide my own furniture. He would charge me £250 a month, which was very cheap for Central London, even in 1993. I gratefully took it on and dubbed it Wuthering Depths.

Thus began my new life. David took on the full-time childcare in my absence, and I continued to be the breadwinner and part-time mother. I loved my job, I loved my children, I loved the countryside and I loved London, but I began to hate my life. On a Sunday evening, the family would drive me down to the station to catch the seven o'clock train, which in principle would have me in London soon after nine.

Unfortunately, not long after, British Rail was taken over by Virgin and train times became outrageously unpredictable. Sometimes the train was so overcrowded that I and a couple of other regular Sunday-nighters would complete the journey in the guard's little compartment at the front of the train. On numerous occasions the service was so late and so poor that we would arrive in Euston at two or three in the morning. Barely time to get to the flat before I had to leave again for work. There'd be horrible sandwiches and a bottle of wine from the buffet to share with the other regulars and, together, we dubbed our weekly experience of travelling 'Virgin on the Ridiculous'.

All my determination to eat wisely, preparing only the very best of good fresh food, fell completely by the wayside. Monday morning came with the usual early start, lattes (two) and croissants (two). Lunch continued in the canteen or the local restaurants and then I would return to my lonely little hole in Camden. I'd have a bit of a sleep in the afternoon, wake around six, call home to check everyone was OK and merely reinforce a terrible sense of loneliness and dislocation.

Of course there were good friends in London, but they were generally occupied with their own families. There'd be the usual occasional trips to the theatre and, as often as possible, dinners with friends around the corner at the Camden Brasserie – famously known to serve the best chips in London and fabulous puddings. They were my greatest pleasures. Even now, nothing delights me more than an evening spent in an excellent restaurant with good friends. Those lovely meals became the highlights of my working week.

When I was alone in Wuthering Depths, which was often – I spent Sunday, Monday, Tuesday and Wednesday nights there – there was one major drawback. The renovated kitchen had no oven. I had a microwave and a gas hob for cooking. I treated myself very badly. I don't recall ever cooking a decent meal there. On a Monday afternoon I would pop down to the local Sainsbury's or Marks & Spencer and fill the fridge with pre-packaged foods. Spaghetti bolognese, spaghetti carbonara, Chinese dishes that could be microwaved – you get the picture. My microbiome must have been screaming at my neglectful failure to provide it with any decent healthy bacteria.

Then, of course, there were takeaways. There was a pizza place nearby and an Indian restaurant. I would phone. They would deliver. There was always a bottle of wine on the go. I'm afraid there were quite a few of us at that time who treated dry white wine as a non-alcoholic drink, and I think that remains the case for a significant number of us – that old 'wine o'clock' thing. How come I didn't have the good sense to realize that, with the croissants, the toast, the sandwiches, the takeaways, the microwaved 'quickies' and the alcohol, my intake of calories was phenomenal?

Actually, I clearly did. I'm not a stupid woman and I had plenty of knowledge about the risks of eating nothing but that which the food industry put on my plate – the salt, the sugar and the preservatives – but I had become so isolated and so miserable I simply used what was undoubtedly tasty food and relaxing booze for comfort. I became the classic comfort eater. No useful bacteria were heading for my gut at all.

We all know how easy it is for our best-laid plans to go

awry. We all experience incredibly stressful periods in our lives. We might change jobs, move house, go through a divorce or find ourselves in that toughest of times – being the filling in life's sandwich, where our teenage children and our elderly parents need us and there's no time to think about ourselves. Food is so often what we turn to for comfort.

On a Thursday afternoon I would fetch up at Euston again, buy a nice French-bread sandwich and another latte and make my way to the train, hoping it would leave on time and get me to Macclesfield as David and the kids turned up to take me home. Bless them, they were always so pleased to see me and never once made any comment about how much weight I seemed to be gaining. I was just lovely, cuddly Mum, and David would have cooked something fresh and delicious for our early-evening meal. I then had Friday, Saturday and most of Sunday to be what and who I wanted to be. A wife and mother, living a healthy lifestyle.

It's strange that I never really became aware of how much fatter I was getting. It's that thing again of looking at yourself in the mirror day after day, doing your hair in much the same way, applying make-up in the style you've always done, wearing the same, loose clothes you've always preferred – I'd never been the kind of follower of fashion who'd go for closely fitting tops, and skirts and tailored jackets. My comfort zone was a pair of stretchy black trousers with a nicely expansive waist and a baggy top to go over them. So, as I looked in the mirror each day, I saw pretty much the same person I'd seen the day before.

I did know I was becoming profoundly depressed, and from time to time it occurred to me that my eating and drinking were in danger of becoming obsessive behaviours. I was too sad to make the effort to do anything about it. Food was pleasure, food was comfort. It had always been so. I was also at that stage when the perimenopause and then the menopause begin to kick in; when I began to wonder if my clothes were getting a little bit tighter than they'd been before, I simply put it down to the inevitability of middle-age spread.

I went to my doctor because I felt so low. I'd known her for a long time and got on very well with her. She never weighed me or ever suggested that I might be getting a little overweight. It's significant, I think, that she too was rather fat. Maybe she should have alerted me to my increasing girth, but she didn't. I guess I comforted myself with the fact that we were both 'big girls' and if she really thought I was going too far she would say something. Instead, she was deeply sympathetic to my depressed state and prescribed Prozac.

It helped a bit, and throughout that period I still managed to be the bright and cheery Jenni Murray who said a welcoming 'good morning' to the radio audience during the week. At the weekends I managed to be 'fun mum', going riding with Ed, cheering on Charlie from the touchline as he developed his skills on the rugby field, and would always be there for the last few hours on a Sunday evening to give whatever help I could with their homework before leaving for the station.

I was reluctant to stay on the anti-depressants for very long. They lifted the terrible low mood I'd been suffering, but somehow felt like a weak cop-out. So, after six months, I weaned myself off them. I went back to the doctor, who confirmed I was clearly perimenopausal – that time of hot flushes, night sweats, irregular and often flooding periods before they finally stop and you can be considered menopausal. Without much discussion, her response to my question about the possibility of HRT was, 'Sure, what do you want? Pills or patches?'

There's been so much discussion in recent years about the safety or otherwise of HRT, so a GP might be a little more cautious these days about offering a prescription so blithely. It's something that's worth having a good discussion about and making an informed decision. After all, it landed me in trouble. When I was diagnosed with breast cancer my consultant oncologist had no doubt about a connection with HRT.

The HRT certainly seemed to give me something of an energy boost, but the depression, the comfort eating and the excessive attachment to a glass of dry white wine began to kick in again. One miserable evening in Wuthering Depths, after a particularly difficult day at the office and worries about money, my parents who were elderly and not very well, deadlines and the kids doing exams, I actually picked up the phone and called the Samaritans. I just needed someone to talk to. Someone who had no idea who I was and to whom I could spill out all my anxieties. I shall always be grateful to the anonymous young man who listened so patiently as I sobbed my heart out.

It was an official 'celebrity' dinner at the newly renovated Café Royal on London's Regent Street that prompted me to think seriously about my weight. I was seated at the top table alongside the paterfamilias of the Forte family, Lord Charles Forte. He couldn't have been more charming, but as we tucked into a delicious meal he looked at me somewhat quizzically and said, 'You know, you really could be a very beautiful young woman, but I think you're becoming too fat.'

I was staggered at such hurtful frankness and spent the rest of the dinner giving rather stiff responses to his attempts at making polite conversation. I honestly don't think he was remotely aware of how rude I thought he'd been. I left in a bit of a huff as soon as the coffee had been served, but his words rankled. I went to John Lewis the very next day and bought weighing scales, something I'd vowed I would never do again, all those years ago when I'd last been obsessed with my size.

What a terrible shock. The scales did not lie. I weighed 16 stone. How come I hadn't been told by my husband or my dearest friends that I had really become quite porky? Were they all just too kind to want to hurt or upset me? Could it be that some of my friends – all lovely and slim – rather liked having a fat friend who made them look even more attractive?

Why hadn't I noticed that whenever we went out to dinner together for one of our immensely pleasurable 'girls' nights out' we all ordered the lovely chips at the Brasserie – a great big bowlful for each person – but Sally or Jane or Norma had merely nibbled at a few and I had scoffed the lot? What was wrong with me? Why had it taken a complete stranger to voice those terrible words that every fat person dreads: 'You know, you could be quite pretty if you lost some weight'?

My first response was to go back to my precious copy of *Fat Is a Feminist Issue*. I wanted to remind myself of the therapeutic approach Susie Orbach and a number of other psychologists had developed to help so many women deal with the obsession with food and weight that occupied much of their time and energy. Fifty per cent of women in the US, she said, were estimated to be overweight. The UK was not far behind. I read her again:

> The fact that compulsive eating is overwhelmingly a woman's problem suggests it has something to do with the experience of being female in our society. Feminism argues that

being fat represents an attempt to break free of society's sex stereotypes. Getting fat can thus be understood as a definite and purposeful act; it is a directed, conscious or unconscious challenge to sex role stereotyping and culturally defined experience of womanhood. Fat is a social disease, and fat is a feminist issue. Fat is not about lack of self-control or lack of willpower. Fat is about protection, sex, nurturance, strength, boundaries, mothering, substance, asserting and rage. Fat expresses experiences of women today in ways that are seldom examined and even more seldom treated . . . What is it about the social position of women that leads them to respond to it by getting fat?

Good grief. Was that what I'd been doing? Filling the holes left by my separation from my family, panicking about being the breadwinner and keeping the whole family afloat financially, raging at my mother's constant emphasis on thinness and attractiveness, and the expectations that had been loaded on me during my career in television, and the perceived assumptions – from my mother, my bosses and my colleagues – that my appearance carried more weight than my brain? I remembered how often my mother said she hadn't really been listening to the scripts I had written or the questions I had posed in interviews, but wanted to talk about the way I looked. Was my weight gain an act of anger and massive defiance? Was getting fat an expression of my feminism, a 'Screw you!' to the expectations attached to being a wife, mother and, in my case, increasingly public figure?

I knew that Susie Orbach and a group of her colleagues had developed a new kind of psychoanalysis, which rejected the classical therapy that had no feminist perspective. She explains in her book that since the Second World War psychiatry had, by and large, no comprehension of the painful and conflicting experiences that feminist thinking had begun to uncover about the way women feel about themselves. Traditional psychotherapy had developed entirely from a male understanding, or lack of understanding, of what women were about. The purpose of the new feminist psychotherapy was, yes, to try to reduce the obesity that resulted from compulsive eating, but, most importantly, to treat the underlying cause of distress that produced it.

Susie has spoken to so many women who have suffered, and has compiled a list of what she has learned defines the problem. So, compulsive eating is:

1. Eating when you are not physically hungry.
2. Feeling out of control around food, submerged by either dieting or gorging.
3. Spending a good deal of time thinking and worrying about food and fatness.
4. Scouring the latest diet for vital information.
5. Feeling awful about yourself as someone who is out of control.
6. Feeling awful about your body.

I got in touch with Susie and went to see her at her practice in North London. We had met a number of times professionally, with me as the interviewer and Susie as the interviewee. It was very strange to find our positions reversed, and we finally agreed that we knew each other too well for Susie to act as my therapist. She referred me to another female psychotherapist who was approved by the Women's Therapy Centre and I began my weekly treatment.

I shan't mention the name of the woman I saw because, for

me, it didn't work. I would turn up at her house at the appointed time, sit in a comfy chair in her treatment room with her sitting opposite me, a table with a box of tissues on it between us, and she would say virtually nothing throughout the hour-long session. It was apparent that I was expected to do the talking. I made it clear that it was being fat that had brought me to her, but I had expected her to question me and perhaps make useful suggestions about how I might resolve some of the questions I was raising. That never happened. I would babble on about what I'd been eating, how I'd been missing the children, something my mother had said, occasionally bursting into tears; and response was there none.

For some people, therapy can be tremendously helpful. We all think we can talk things over with our friends, but there will be occasions when they don't have the time or patience to take on our problems. Equally, we may need to discuss things more deeply and share more than we might want to with friends, and a stranger who's trained to be objective, ask the right questions and listen well can be the right way to go. It's best to be wary, though, and make sure the therapist is the best one for you.

In my case, as the hour came to a close, this woman simply said the session was over and she would see me the following week. I would hand over fifty quid, leave and find somewhere to have a cup of coffee and a bun! Not quite the object of the exercise. I stuck with it for a few weeks, maybe even a few months, but I know that I eventually went into performance mode, trying to get some response out of her. I would tell what I thought were amusing stories that had happened at work, maybe relate a few jokes or a bit of gossip I'd picked up. There was no response, never so much as a smile, and no advice to tell me to stop trying to entertain her and take the whole business seriously. Finally, I quit. What was the point of me paying her to entertain her? I guess psychotherapy was not for me.

Neither, as it turned out, was cognitive behavioural therapy. A friend of mine who'd had a very bad car accident in which the other person involved had been seriously injured – not my friend's fault – had suffered terrible depression as a result and found CBT tremendously helpful. It's a therapy that claims to help you understand the impact your thoughts have on the way you feel and behave, and teaches you to 'create more helpful thinking patterns and healthier behaviours'. I tried it. Frankly, I was ready to grasp at any straw. I was getting fatter. I didn't speak to any family or friends about my sense of desperation. I was heading towards fifty and, given my vow never to go on a diet again, I had no idea how to reduce my burgeoning waistline if my brain was continuing to tell me that having something nice to eat would make me feel better.

The second woman I saw didn't appear to have heard the word 'feminism', and hadn't much of a clue about Orbach's theories on the reasons for compulsive and comfort eating. I recall her advising me to think happy thoughts when the sadness or anxiety engulfed me, and to start thinking about food as a necessary fuel rather than as a pleasure or a comfort. I saw her a few times, did the homework she set me to try to alter my thinking on fatness and food (there's a whole trend these days that suggests you can 'think yourself thin' – you can't) and I didn't stick with CBT for very long.

These talking therapies work for some people, but for me they were just something else filling up my already overstretched schedule. I did the inevitable, broke the promise I'd made to myself all those years ago at university, and turned to a diet.

5

The Best-laid Plans

In the mid-1990s, copies of *The Atkins Diet* were literally flying off the shelves. I bought a copy. It was described as a keto diet. I hadn't a clue what that meant, so, naturally, looked it up. Ketones are acids produced when the body burns its own fat. The chemicals are made in the liver when you don't have enough insulin in your body to turn sugar, or glucose, into energy. High-carbohydrate diets raise blood sugar levels, which in turn signal the body to secrete more insulin. The body creates more fat and your metabolism adjusts itself to burn sugar. The Atkins diet restricts foods that raise blood sugars and insulin – carbohydrates.

You need another source of energy when there's no sugar or carbs to provide it, so the body burns fat instead. The liver turns the fat into ketones and sends them into your bloodstream. It sounded simple enough and burning fat was exactly what I was after, but changing the body's chemistry and creating a state called ketosis, I thought, must come with some sort of risk. Indeed it does, particularly if you're diabetic, which I'm not.

For type 1 diabetics it can cause an unsafe level of ketosis, which can result in diabetic ketoacidosis and a coma, requiring emergency medical treatment. Because the body is not producing its own insulin, its muscles and fat stores are unable to absorb any glucose, uncontrolled amounts of ketones are produced and only fat is burned. Dr Giles Yeo, the Cambridge geneticist who specializes in the science of obesity, says in his book, *Gene Eating*, that 'this, by the way, is my riposte to those who say we can live perfectly healthy lives without any carbohydrates and just use ketones from the breakdown of fat as fuel. Without at least some carbohydrates in our diet, we would die.'

It's said to be unlikely for a non-diabetic to reach life-threatening levels of ketosis, but there is a good deal of scientific controversy about the high-fat, low-carb protein plan recommended by Atkins. A number of clinicians, like Dr Yeo, regard eliminating carbohydrates as unhealthy and dangerous. The Atkins book does recommend regular testing of the urine to indicate whether or not a safe level of ketosis has been achieved. You dip a test strip into a fresh urine specimen and the colour to which the tip changes indicates the level of ketosis reached. Bit of a pain, frankly, but I did it religiously. There was one problem with the regime. My breath smelled like nail-varnish remover. When your body is in a state of ketosis there's a breakdown of acetoacetic acid into acetone and carbon dioxide, which you exhale.

There are other unpleasant side effects to contend with, depending on how strictly you try to stick to a high-protein and low-carb regime. Heart palpitations, headaches, cramps in the legs, constipation and bad breath are all reported as common. From time to time during the diet I suffered them all.

The Atkins diet is divided into four phases – induction, ongoing weight loss, pre-maintenance and maintenance – but effectively you're eating a lot of protein, very little carbohydrate and a whole lot of fat. On any ketogenic diet you're consuming 75–80 per cent fat – butter, the fatty bit on the grilled lamb chop, bacon and egg for breakfast, and if you're a yogurt fan, you never buy any that claims to be fat-free. Your protein consumption, as calories have to come from somewhere, can be as high as 25 per cent, compared to the 15 per cent found in the typical Western diet of the twenty-first century.

Following the diet to the letter was arduous and my family thought I was nuts. No bread, no pasta, no rice, no buns, no cakes, no biscuits, no potatoes, no sweetcorn, no apples or bananas – so many of my favourite things were totally off the menu. Of course I bought them for the rest of the family and it took every ounce of my limited self-control to resist the occasional cheat. But resist I did.

It was necessary to measure absolutely everything in the four phases the diet demands. You have to lower your carb intake to 20–40 grams a day to achieve ketosis and you have to get those carbs from nutrient-rich, non-starchy sources. You're told that 12–15 grams of those carbs have to come from 'foundation vegetables' – anything from asparagus through to broccoli, spinach and lettuce was allowed, but only in small portions. Fruits were allowed, but only the low-glycaemic varieties such as blackberries, raspberries and tomatoes. Tomatoes, of course, are technically fruits.

Protein had to make up 20–30 per cent of the diet and you were allowed four 170-gram servings each day. Bacon and eggs for breakfast was always a good option, but I did start to grow worried when dietary warnings about a possible carcinogenic connection with processed meats began to filter through, information about which is constantly changing. Just eggs, then! A small steak fried in olive oil with some broccoli became my regular dinner, and lunch might have been a bit of fish or some prawns with a salad. Cheese and yogurt were allowed, but because cheese contains about a gram of carbs per 28 grams you were only allowed around 13 grams per day. Twenty-eight grams was about the size of a 2.5-centimetre cube. Surprisingly for a weight-loss diet, fat consumption was encouraged. It was recommended that 60 per cent of your daily calories should come from any fats, apart, of course, from the trans fats found in packaged and fried foods. The recommended daily intake of fats such as sesame, walnut or olive oils was 2–4 tablespoons.

Some nuts and seeds were allowed as a snack, but my favourites – cashews, pine, almonds and pistachios – were to be avoided as they contain more carbs than, say, hazelnuts, pecans, sunflower seeds or walnuts. Plenty of water was recommended to prevent dizziness, and fizzy drinks with zero calories were allowed. Again, I worried about the consumption of diet drinks. Concerns about artificial sweeteners such as aspartame were beginning to be voiced, so I cut them out. Adding extra salt was advised to provide electrolytes. I'm not at all sure diet drinks or extra salt can be considered healthy additions to a diet, particularly for anyone with high blood pressure or a heart condition. Booze, of course, was right off the menu.

Pure alcohol, at 7 calories per gram, contains almost the same number of calories as fat, which has 9 calories per gram. All alcoholic drinks, whether beer, wine, gin or whisky, are equally calorific. A 175-millilitre glass of wine with an alcohol content of 13 per cent contains nearly 160 calories, and a whole bottle contains around 700 calories. A standard 330-millilitre bottle of beer with 5 per cent alcohol contains 140 calories. A pint in the pub is more than 140 calories. Then there are the alcopops, mixers and other alcoholic drinks that have a high sugar content. You could, on an evening out, consume 700–1,000 calories, which, even if you weren't trying to reduce your weight and were consuming the recommended 2,000 calories for women and 2,500 for men, would mean half your daily amount was taken up by nothing more than a few drinks.

It kind of puts the fashionable idea of 'wine o'clock' into perspective and confirms what my friend Sally and I always used to say to each other as our inhibitions diminished when we frequently shared a bottle of wine. 'How about the five most dangerous words in the English language?' Those five words were 'Shall we open another bottle?' It's also worth bearing in mind the advice given by the former chief medical officer for England, Professor Dame Sally Davies. Pointing out the established connection between excessive alcohol consumption and breast cancer, she warned, 'Think of cancer every time you open a bottle of wine.'

Gosh, it was hard. Proponents of the regime say that on Atkins you never feel hungry or deprived, balancing all these proteins, fats and vegetables. I felt both, all the time, but comforted myself with the loss of a couple of stone in around a year, which took me down to 14 stone. Still technically obese, completely fed up with all the urine testing, and envying friends and family who were tucking in to all the goodies I was missing. That is the life of a dieter. I felt excluded from the pleasures of sharing a lovely meal and it wasn't long before I started to feel really hungry almost all of the time. I tried not to stray from the allowed foods, but my portion sizes began to creep up and it wasn't long before the odd chip started to find its way on to my plate, or a slice of buttered toast after the bacon and eggs. It was, in the end, simply unsustainable and my weight began, again, to creep up. There's much to say about why these diets rarely work as a long-term solution. It's the brain, obviously, and we'll come back to the part the head plays in all this in Chapter 8.

By the time we reached the millennium, my weight gain was considerable and I was about to enter the worst decade of my life. I was still travelling up and down the West Coast Main Line, spending the week in Wuthering Depths and supporting one seventeen-year-old through his A levels in subjects of which I had zero understanding – physics, biology and chemistry. He was intent on entering university to study veterinary medicine and the other son, four years behind him, was playing a lot of rugby and heading towards GCSEs. At least I could help with his chosen favourite subjects of French, English and history, but at weekends I spent an awful lot of time cheering from the touchline at venues across the North West.

Hot dogs with sugary ketchup became a frequent Sunday lunch after matches. Delicious but disastrous. Dr Giles Yeo has a word of warning about ketchup. He claims that if you consume only an extra 7 calories a day for thirty years you will gain 2½ stone in that period. When he asked himself what 7 calories look like, he found a bottle of ketchup. The nutritional information on the bottle said a 'serving' of ketchup is 15 grams. Even such a small portion – and I suspect we all squeeze on more – would amount to 15 calories. Calculated over thirty years, with a dollop every day, the weight gain would be nearly 5 stone. Scary!

Meanwhile, my mother's Parkinson's had taken a terrifying hold on her, physically and mentally. Dad had developed an alarming cough and was finding caring for her an increasingly onerous task. As their only child I was the sole person, with David and the boys' assistance, to give them any support.

There's no doubt that the middle years, when we might expect to slow down a bit, are the most hectic for so many of us. Lots of us have had our children later than used to be common, but they continue to need our attention throughout their teenage years. We might have established jobs or careers, have ageing parents who need assistance, and we are, quite simply, constantly busy. We grab a sandwich here and there, maybe order in a takeaway or cook something that's quick and easy – spag bol or chilli con carne again. And maybe we can be forgiven for searching for the occasional treat to relax us. A glass of wine, a comforting latte in the morning, a bag of sweets in the car. We seem so often to be living in a world that's all about work, earning to pay the mortgage, getting the kids the nice clothes and trainers they long for. Is it any wonder we seek release from stress at every turn?

I was spending part of every weekend crossing the Pennines to my parents' home in Barnsley to make sure they had plenty of food in the house and to help Dad cook it. An alarming number of weekdays were spent negotiating with doctors and social workers to try to achieve some sort of respite care for Dad in their home or for a short time in a care home. I was generally unsuccessful, it has to be said, and Dad was determined Mum should not leave the house for permanent care. He wasn't worried about having to pay for it, although he shouldn't have had to even think of it as she was often so terribly ill; he just wanted them to stay together in their home for as long as was possible.

Even though my mother's usual frankness about my size never waned – every visit began with the familiar 'Ooh, love, you've put some more on. You must do something about it. You look awful' – my anxiety about getting bigger and bigger went to the bottom of my agenda. I fooled around a bit on my own with more silly diets. I even managed a few days on the revolting cabbage soup one, but the comfort of something delicious – and plenty of it – felt like the only pleasure available to me.

In 2006 it all came to a head. My mother, finally, had to be admitted to a care home and my father spent every minute of every day by her side. As I became fatter and fatter, she became dangerously emaciated. Parkinson's ends when the patient can no longer swallow, and towards Christmas of 2006 she reached that point. I, meanwhile, suffered the fate of so many women who've put on excessive amounts of weight and continued to treat dry white wine as a non-alcoholic drink. In the shower, I found my right breast had an inverted nipple. I knew what it meant.

I went to the GP, who rushed me off to have a biopsy. I was on the way to see my consultant surgeon to have my diagnosis of breast cancer confirmed when my phone rang. My mother had died that night. Without doubt it was the worst day of my life.

I have no truck with those people who have complained about the Cancer Research UK ads that show a cigarette box with the words 'obesity is a cause of cancer' displayed on the front. It's a powerful way of expressing the fact that when it comes to certain cancers, including liver, ovarian and breast, obesity presents as much of a risk as smoking. Whilst I have already stated that I abhor fat shaming when 'fat cow' and 'fat bitch' are called out in the street – or when people are told 'you're a greedy pig' or 'it's easy, just eat less and exercise more' – it is ridiculous to accuse a serious charity, basing its advertising on rigorous scientific research, of fat shaming. I know to my cost that what that advert is warning us about is absolutely true. In 2018, only 14 per cent of adults in the UK were smokers but 26 per cent of British adults were classed as obese, according to Public Health England and the Office for National Statistics. Our cancer rates keep on rising, despite the reduction in the numbers of those who smoke.

Smoking is incredibly difficult to quit, as is the kind of eating disorder that leads to obesity. It's a disorder some would call a disease. Debatable, but I would go along with the idea that if disease is understood literally, dis-ease is exactly what you feel when you're fat. Nor must we forget that obesity and smoking are more prevalent among the poorest in our society than the better off, and we must have sympathy and understanding, and make help available, for those who struggle. But it makes no sense at all to conceal the facts on which we can all base our choices and our efforts to try to save our health and, in some cases, our lives.

Christmas was awful that year. We had to wait to arrange my mother's funeral as nothing could be done during the long holiday. On the other hand, my surgeon wanted to operate as soon as possible. I was admitted to Manchester's Christie Hospital the day after Boxing Day and my only comforting thought was that my mother had never had to know I had the disease she had dreaded for most of her adult life. The days between Christmas and New Year were spent recuperating from the mastectomy, and the moment I was allowed to go home I was crossing the Pennines again to support my father and deliver the eulogy at my mother's funeral.

For the next few months, life could not have been harder. I had to continue to work through the chemotherapy – we needed the money. My father's dreadful cough turned out to be advanced lung cancer and he died peacefully in the wonderful hospice in Barnsley in the early part of June that year. Both my parents had lived to the age of eighty and whilst I grieved terribly for them, feeling like a lonely, only orphan at the age of fifty-seven, there was a sense of relief that their suffering was over. My mother had devoted her life to cooking and caring for us in the best way she could to keep us fit and healthy, but they had both had painful and miserable final years. Even with their best efforts at taking care of our diet and never falling into a fondness for alcohol – my parents barely drank at all – the luck of the health draw is just that, a lucky draw, and they were not winners in the lottery.

I tried, as always, to joke my way through my own difficulties. Early in the cancer treatment I managed to upset friends and family by saying losing a breast was great – it would knock a few pounds off the scales. Then I would quote an old friend, Liz Tilberis, who'd been the editor of *Vogue* and then *Harper's Bazaar*. Liz had been diagnosed with ovarian cancer and died in 1999. In her days at *Vogue* she'd often laughed about being a very average size 14 and unable to fit into any of the fabulous but unreasonably tiny fashion samples that came into her office. As the cancer took its toll she lost a considerable amount of weight. 'Fantastic,' she told me, 'this cancer diet works. You should try it!'

Unfortunately, the cancer diet didn't work for me. It might seem a little crazy even to have considered it might be a good idea. Of course, I was kind of trying to find something to laugh about in even suggesting it might be a useful way to lose weight, but I also suspect my attitude smacked of a degree of desperation. How could I have even considered that a disease that might kill me and the surgical mutilation of my body was better than being fat?

More than half of women with breast cancer experience weight gain during treatment, according to the American Society of Clinical Oncology. Obviously, being overweight before treatment begins doesn't help, but chemotherapy and steroids often contribute to weight gain rather than the loss you might expect. Chemotherapy can cause the body to hold on to excess fluid, the exhaustion it causes leads to a considerable reduction in physical activity, and when you feel sick after the horrible chemicals have been streamed into your body the best way to get rid of the nausea is to eat. I remember my husband picking me up after my first, terrifying dose. I felt sick and, at the same time, ravenously hungry.

He took me straight away to a favourite Argentinian steak house in Manchester where I consumed a huge steak, chips, veg and a delicious chocolate pudding. I no longer felt nauseated, but, even after all that, I still felt hungry! Chemotherapy is known to trigger intense food cravings. I'm not really that much of a chocolate fan, but I developed a passion for Twixes and Maltesers. Another unwanted side effect of the treatment is often a change in the patient's metabolism. Your body loses much of its ability to utilize its energy. Fatal for someone who puts on weight as easily as I do.

Then there are the steroids prescribed to reduce swelling and pain, to treat the nausea and, sometimes, as part of the treatment for the cancer itself. Common side effects of steroids are an increase in appetite and a development of extra fatty tissue, which can cause your stomach to swell and your face and neck to blow up in size. Of course, I got the lot!

The doctors who were responsible for my ongoing treatment at the Nightingale Centre in Manchester had begun working on a new kind of diet for their breast-cancer patients to try to deal with these problems. They also hoped it would become a popular and well-known diet that might help women to lose weight early enough to decrease the risk of developing breast cancer. It was refined and promoted by Dr Michael Mosley as the 5:2 diet and became enormously popular. It involves eating normally for five days of the week, preferably following a Mediterranean diet of fish, meat, olive oil, a range of vegetables and plenty of fruit and tomatoes, then for two days a week you fast, eating only 500 calories a day. A generous portion of vegetables is allowed on the fasting days, together with natural yogurt and berries but no sugar or honey, boiled or baked eggs, grilled fish or lean meat, cauliflower rice, low-calorie soups and black coffee. Professor Tim Spector, the genetic epidemiologist and author of *The Diet Myth*, is, obviously, generally not a fan of dieting, but does say that the 5:2, if carried out to the letter, with a wide range of fresh foods providing the microbes the gut needs to function correctly, is the only diet that he would recommend. But, like any diet, it needs to be sustained.

I tried very hard with the fasting diet whilst the chemotherapy continued. Then, when it was over some six months later, I vowed to be kind to myself and bring my burgeoning weight down by sticking to the regime. I managed it during treatment, in the latter part of the three-week chemo cycle, just as I was starting to feel human again after the latest hit. I made a real effort to eat according to 5:2 principles, knowing my body needed to be as strong and fit as possible to withstand the onslaught of the chemotherapy.

I did my fasting on days when I was at work and had only myself to think of, then ate whatever the family was having on other days. I stuck mainly with fruit and veg on fast days and aimed to keep down portions on other days, but the drugs made it hard as I was so often so hungry and found it difficult to go through such a miserable time without the occasional sweet treat, croissant or sandwich.

The treatment plan meant going to the hospital on a Thursday afternoon after I'd finished work, sitting in one of the big comfy chairs in the unit and having a cannula stuck into a vein in my left hand. I had had a right-breast mastectomy, so no injections or pricks of any kind were allowed in my right hand or arm. A couple of the lymph nodes in my right armpit had been removed during the surgery as a preventative measure to stop the cancer spreading. It means my right arm and hand could be prone to infection from now on.

The drugs were delivered in the same place at the same time every three weeks. For a week after a dose I would feel absolutely ghastly – nauseated, hungry and exhausted. In the second week I would begin to feel a little more human, and by the third week I would feel absolutely fine and strong enough, physically and emotionally, to discipline my diet. I wasn't consistent enough in my endeavours for any loss of weight to be achieved, but I convinced myself I was being positive, making an effort, and would be able to take myself completely in hand once the regular chemotherapy was over.

It was not to be. A few weeks after my treatment ended and I was beginning to feel fitter and reconciled to my mutilated body, I began to experience a pain in my right hip. I ignored it, thinking I must have slept in an awkward position or maybe had twisted it scurrying up or down the stairs to Wuthering Depths. It didn't go away. In fact it got worse, much worse, and every step I took became agony. I couldn't even find a comfortable position in which to sleep. Still I tried to ignore it until, some weeks later, my left hip began to feel painful too.

'OK,' I thought, 'you're fifty-seven years old, maybe it's normal for the hips to start to cause trouble as you age.' But the trouble got worse. I bought a stick and tried to manage a normal life. I couldn't. I bought a pair of stylish black crutches, still trying to tell myself it would get better, refusing to accept that being as fat as I was might be putting a serious amount of strain on my joints.

I remember one evening when I had been asked to go to an art gallery in Central London to present an award in a painting competition. I managed to drag myself there, asked for a seat from which to make a little speech, stood up to present the award, refused any of the organizers' generous hospitality and got into a taxi as fast as I could to get myself home and to my bed. I was truly suffering agonizing, almost unbearable pain. Every step I took felt as if my femur and my hip bone were grinding together.

It was a fine night and still not completely dark when I reached the flat. I stood at the top of the stairs, weeping in anticipation of having to descend them. I took out my phone and called my surgical oncologist, Professor Nigel Bundred. He'd been kind enough to give me his mobile number in case of emergency. He answered immediately and I told him about my hips. Could this sudden onset of agony be connected to the cancer or the chemotherapy? 'Ah,' he said. 'I don't want to do a diagnosis over the phone, but it sounds to me as if it might be avascular necrosis. I'll refer you to an orthopaedic surgeon.'

I had never heard of avascular necrosis. Here's what I read when I googled it: 'Avascular necrosis of the femoral head is a pathologic process that results from interruption of the blood supply to the bone. AVN of the hip is poorly understood, but this process is the final common pathway of traumatic or non-traumatic factors that compromise the already precarious circulation of the femoral head. It can lead to tiny breaks of the bone and the bone's eventual collapse.'

The most common causes are thought to be an injury to the bone (which I hadn't had), alcoholism (which I didn't think could be the cause as, although I enjoyed my wine, it was not to a dangerous extent), deep-sea diving and getting the bends coming to the surface (which I had never done), or corticosteroids (which I *had* taken in recent months) and certain cancer treatments, including radiation and chemotherapy.

So that's why my consultant reached his conclusion so quickly. I don't remember being told about this kind of complication, but when I thought about it, I knew of a number of other people who had suffered hip problems after their cancer treatments. I never found out why patients were not warned that something so awful could come as a result of trying to get rid of any residual cancer cells in the body. I guess the oncologist is primarily concerned with delivering the best treatment that's likely to save your life. Maybe they worry that explaining you might have to undergo a bilateral hip replacement only a year after a mastectomy might deter you from going ahead with it.

What happened next meant all my good intentions of sticking with the fasting diet, getting back on an exercise bike, making the effort to go to the pool two or three times a week, and returning to the habit of good long walks in the park in London and the Peak District at home had to be put on hold. I certainly wouldn't be horse riding again. Number-one priority was getting these wretched hips dealt with.

Yet again my promises to take myself in hand and concentrate on getting fitter were abandoned. I knew in my heart that my weight had contributed to both the cancer and the hips, but I had consistently found excuses for not taking more care of myself long before these disasters struck, whether it was diet or exercise. Too busy, too tired, hated the gym, couldn't be bothered, loved to eat – the list is endless. Why is it so common for so many of us to pay ourselves so little attention and risk our strength and health whilst we still have them? Life will always put other priorities in our way, but it's worth bearing in mind that prevention is generally preferable to cure. Now I was not making excuses. I literally could not physically manage to take good care of myself. I could barely stand, let alone walk.

I went for X-rays and an MRI, and the diagnosis was confirmed. Both hips would need to be completely replaced and, in order to enable me to carry on working and moving around, they should be done as quickly as possible to prevent any further deterioration, which could lead to the collapse of the bones. I begged to have both hips replaced on the same day.

I spent a surprisingly comfortable night after the op and don't remember any pain at all. I woke early, was attended to by the nursing staff, given a decent breakfast and then the door to my room opened. In walked two people, one male and one female, who I can only describe as 'strapping'.

'Morning,' they chimed brightly. 'Righty-ho, up you get!'

'Oh no,' said I. 'Don't be ridiculous. It was only yesterday I had both my hips replaced.'

'We know that.' They smiled. 'We're the physios and it's our job to have you walking today and going up and down the stairs before the week's out.'

They were serious. They stood at the side of the bed to support me as I swung my legs towards them. I held on to them and then to the walking frame before taking my first hesitant steps with two completely artificial hips. I was astonished and thrilled. I felt no pain at all.

In less than a week I had learned how to manage the stairs, and that's when David was allowed to collect me and take me home. I slid carefully into the passenger seat, taking care not to dislocate the hips, and from the back seat he brought our little Chihuahua puppy, Butch. A silly name for such a tiny dog, I know, but it had been David's little joke when we first went to pick him from the litter. Butch was so pleased to see me after my absence. I knew I would have a constant companion during my recovery and a powerful motivation to lure me out to the hills, which would get me fit and keep him that way.

The results of the surgery were nothing short of miraculous. I remained free of any pain and a few weeks of physiotherapy in the local swimming pool soon had everything working perfectly. I began to walk Butch with relative ease, being slightly more careful over the bumpy hills of the Peaks than I might have been before, full of fear that I might fall and damage the new hips. All went well and I began to work again, cutting down my working week a little. I now presented *Woman's Hour* for three rather than four days a week. Nevertheless, it was back to the twice-weekly train trips and days spent in Wuthering Depths.

Butch became my companion both in London and at home. I hated leaving him in the flat by himself during the hours I was at Broadcasting House and he hated being left alone. There was only one solution. Get another dog who would keep him company when I couldn't be there. Enter Frieda, and now I had two little créatures entirely dependent on me for their welfare and exercise. But, of course, they're Chihuahuas and very, very small. If the chance of a long and demanding walk came up they were perfectly happy to trot along, but once I was back in the routine of constant travelling, early mornings, resting in the late afternoon and reading piles of books, carrying out research and writing my own books, my former sedentary lifestyle began again. On the whole, they were perfectly happy with a short trot around the neighbourhood and playing in the garden. The weight was creeping up again.

The next step in the cycle of my yo-yo dieting came about as a result of interviewing on *Woman's Hour* the designer of the next trendy, faddy diet. His name was Dr Pierre Dukan. Why, when I had already failed to keep off the weight lost on the Atkins diet and, in fact, had become even fatter than before I'd started on it, was I seduced enough to begin again on a regime that was not all that different from Atkins?

Well, Dr Dukan was French, dapper and extremely charming, and part of my love for France was the language, which I'd studied and spoke fluently, and their passion for delicious food. I couldn't imagine that a Frenchman would possibly seek to deprive any of his followers of their pleasure in eating. Maybe I was too charmed or just too stupid, or maybe I was desperate to find a solution to my weight, which had now increased to 19 stone. Did it not occur to me that the Dukan diet was remarkably similar to Atkins, except there was no mention of ketones and no instruction to test your urine on a regular basis? In September 2010 I began.

As with Atkins there are four phases to the diet. ATTACK (and yes, it's always written in capital letters) is said to give your weight loss a jump start. The second phase is the CRUISE, which supposedly gets you down to your target weight – mine was 12 stone, which I thought a reasonable weight for a woman of 5 foot 7 who'd just turned sixty. The third phase is CONSOLIDATION, which tries to prevent any immediate rebound, and the final phase is STABILIZATION, said to be a long-term strategy to keep the weight off.

Dukan argues that he will redesign your eating habits and help you stabilize your weight for the rest of your life. The diet, though, like Atkins, is extremely restrictive. You're told, in those capitals again, that you can EAT AS MUCH AS YOU LIKE, but your food choices are limited. In effect, it's even more limited than Atkins as the foods included in the hundred on the list are only proteins and low-carb vegetables. Atkins includes fat; Dukan doesn't. He also recommends stirring a tablespoon of oatbran into some fat-free plain yogurt every day. It's supposed to lower your cholesterol.

This time I was determined to be successful, lose the weight, get to where I wanted to be and sustain the diet for ever. This time I would not allow myself to relax and slide back into old habits after I'd lost the weight. I even agreed to write a regular column for the *Daily Mail*, charting my progress. By March 2011 I had lost 3 stone and was looking forward to taking off in October to join my family for the Rugby World Cup in New Zealand – no excess baggage allowed.

I couldn't wait to fly without having to ask for an extension for my safety belt during the flight. (Yes, that had happened to me frequently in the past and there are few things I can think of that are more humiliating than a super-slim flight attendant nodding rather superciliously as you mumble your request for a fat person's strap.) In the article of that date I confessed to having had a bit of a lapse during the CRUISE phase of the diet and gone back to ATTACK – nothing but lean protein and the lightest of green veg and salad.

By early summer I had lost 4 stone and discovered unforeseen consequences to the weight-loss lark. In addition to the pounds from around my waist, I had also lost four items of jewellery, which were irreplaceably valuable. My grandmother's wedding ring had fitted fat me perfectly, as we had our girth in common, and my father had given me my mother's wedding, engagement and eternity rings on her death. She had worn them for sixty years and never removed her wedding ring. They were fine for my little finger.

I had been washing my hands in the bathroom. There was a clatter and a clang, and I watched as the fast-running water took my precious rings in its clutches and washed them down the plughole. I howled in despair and brought David upstairs. He looked desperately anxious, but when he realized what had happened was curiously unsympathetic.

'You should have been more careful. You must have known what would happen. You've lost so much weight.' He gazed at the sink with that resigned 'I could sort it if I had time, being a total expert in all matters DIY, which clearly you are not' look that so many men adopt to make women feel doubly stupid and incompetent.

I burst into tears. 'But they're so precious. Where can they be?' I whined.

'In the S-bend if you're lucky, or in the septic tank if you're not, because in that case you'll never retrieve them because I'm not going there and I doubt you even know where it is! I'll do it on Wednesday.'

It was Sunday. I couldn't bear to think they might be gone and never twinkle on a woman's finger again. It had been my intention to hand them on to my sons to give to the women with whom they choose to share their lives. They could not be allowed to swim about in some revolting mess, never to be retrieved. I begged. He finally took out his tools and to my huge relief found them lodged in the S-bend. I cleaned them and put them away safely. I didn't want to have them altered to fit my thinner fingers. I guess I knew myself well enough to suspect they may not remain this thin for ever.

Traci Mann, Professor of Psychology at the University of Minnesota and author of *Secrets from the Eating Lab*, having reviewed every trial of diets that included one of at least two years, found dieters lost weight in the first nine to twelve months, but over the next two to five years regained all but an average of 2.1 pounds. It's reckoned anything between 80 and 97 per cent of us will regain almost all the weight lost, and significant numbers will become fatter than they were before the diet. I guess it's why my wardrobe, and those of so many of us, have 'thin' clothes and 'fat' clothes so there's always something that will fit.

Yet I persevered with the Dukan diet with very few lapses. One came when David and I had been to see *The King's Speech* at the cinema and were starving afterwards. We stopped for a pizza. (I know!) 'Are you allowed to eat pizza?' he said suddenly. 'Allowed? *Allowed?* Of course I am, if I want to!' He said no more, but was clearly confused that after months of demanding that he put no rice or potatoes on my plate, avoid buying beans, peas, cakes or biscuits, keep the bread out of my way and the dressing away from salad, here I was merrily munching away at the delicious crispy crust. Guilt meant I gave him three-quarters of mine. How come he could eat one and three-quarter pizzas and not put on an ounce? Not fair. But all very well explained by science, which we'll come to later on.

As the fat continued to fall away with, on the whole, careful attention to every mouthful, the scales had begun to welcome me every morning as I approached them, rather than looking fearful that I might crush them under my weight. But inevitably further tests of resolve loomed. The first was my second son Charlie's graduation ceremony at Liverpool University. Champagne was, of course, an inevitability, and along with lots of other parents and their children we went for lunch at the Philharmonic Dining Rooms, arguably the most beautiful pub in England.

I had everything planned to conform with the diet, always a necessary process for the dieter who knows she's going to eat out and has to plan to eat only in restaurants where there'll be low-calorie food on the menu. Scouse, that Liverpool staple of stewed meat, potatoes and pickled red cabbage on the side, would be fine as long as I fished out the potatoes. To my horror, when we arrived I found scouse was no longer on the menu – a discovery I described as an unforgivable flouting of culinary history. My eating plan was scuppered and the only thing on the menu that I could adapt was a fish-finger sandwich with chips.

I didn't eat the bread or the chips and, of course, the fish fingers – fancifully advertised as goujons – didn't fit the diet either as the breadcrumbs coating the fish, the fat in which they were fried and the smidgeon of tomato ketchup into which I dipped them to make them remotely edible were far from Dukan-friendly. I spent the entire graduation ceremony perched high in a far-too-narrow seat at the top of the city's Philharmonic Hall, cheering for my son, mopping up the tears of pride at his success but feeling hunger pangs tugging at my stomach.

Another totally unexpected lure to default on the diet came in August as a result of the fruit-and-vegetable garden we had established a couple of years earlier, which was now producing its first luscious harvest. There was, of course, no problem with the rocket, spinach, tomatoes and cabbages, and I didn't get too concerned about eschewing the potatoes that were growing like weeds but were, according to head gardener David, the most delicious varieties he'd ever tasted, whether roasted, baked, mashed, duchesse or chipped. Of course, I just told myself I wasn't bothered, but I was, in fact, unsurprisingly annoyed and maniacally jealous as he cooked them beautifully and loaded them on to his plate. I still resisted.

It's all tough and a huge test of self-control, but the thing that drove me almost mad with unsatisfied longing was the fruit, which at every turn said 'Eat Me'. As a child I used to weed for my grandfather and got paid a penny a bucket and as many raspberries, strawberries, blackberries and gooseberries as I could eat on the job. Now I was still doing the weeding and the picking but with no pay and no pleasure of consumption, as fruit was still banned from the ATTACK phase of the diet.

What was even worse was David's discovery of the delights of jam-making. I would come into the kitchen to the fragrant aroma of raspberries bubbling away in one pot and rhubarb, gooseberries and ginger in another. Both, of course, loaded with sugar. Some of the finished product was already set and stored in Kilner jars. Whilst I restricted myself to eggs, eggs or eggs and black coffee for breakfast, I would have to endure David whizzing up the milk for a full-fat latte and slathering lashings of butter on several slices of toast whilst extolling the virtues of perfect, home-grown, home-made preserves.

I managed to stick with my resolve to send money to charities helping to feed starving children in Somalia, appeals for which were appearing daily on the television. In the face of terrible hunger in so many parts of the world it seemed obscene to be moaning about what I was not allowed to consume. I am often struck by how disgusting our Western eating disorders are. Whether we're overeaters, anorexics or bulimics, we hardly have the right to indulge in the neurosis of plenty when so many have absolutely nothing to eat. Even those of us who don't have an eating disorder have no difficulty filling our supermarket trolleys and fridges with far more food than we need and then blithely throwing it away when it goes out of date. It's shocking.

I persevered throughout the summer, still picturing myself jumping on that plane to New Zealand and fitting comfortably into the seat and the safety belt. After a year of Dukan and having graduated to the CRUISE phase, which allowed some fruits, but was still lean, grilled protein and low-carb veg, I had not quite made it to my target of 12 stone. However, the 19 stone had gone down to 13 stone 10 pounds and I was feeling so much healthier and pleased with myself. I lumbered less and even managed stairs without feeling like I would die halfway up. I came to the conclusion, as I wrote my final progress report for the *Mail*, that as long as you're ruthlessly strict with yourself, Dukan works brilliantly. Even if you're as weak-willed as me it works pretty well too. That's high praise in the world of diets and, for a while, I genuinely believed this.

There's no doubt I would have lost more weight had there not been the occasional lapses. I had so enjoyed the bronzed roasted potatoes (only one!) and the plum pudding and brandy sauce in which I'd indulged at Christmas. There'd also been one occasion when a little voice had whispered in my ear, 'Go on, Mum, a bit of treacle sponge and custard won't do you any harm!'

I had expected to make changes to my wardrobe as the pounds fell away. My options would widen as my frame narrowed. I found, though, that I disliked shopping as much as ever and stuck with the style I'd developed for an easy sartorial life. I continued to wear the baggy block tops and stretchy trousers with an elasticated waist, and built a collection of colourful scarves to add some brightness and conceal the slightly lopsided post-mastectomy look. I was comfortable and still found not having to make decisions about what to wear every morning so much easier.

My friend Sally had often tried to get me interested in fashion, but I'd always resisted her attempts to lure me to the shops. It's partly that fear of embarrassment in communal changing rooms again, and of sniffy shop assistants convinced nothing they have will fit you. There's also, I think, to some degree, an element of defiance aimed towards my mother. To her, clothes really mattered and she wanted me to share her passion. I quite deliberately never did, because the way she wanted me to look – smart stuff, twin sets and pearls – was not me at all.

The family had gone off to New Zealand early for the start of the Rugby World Cup and it had been much easier to stick to the diet in their absence. There was little call for elaborately cooked meals and no carbohydrates passed through the door, let alone across my lips. Only one hiccup occurred when Charlie, now a photographer, won a UK Picture Editors' Guild Award and, in his absence, I was asked to go to the black-tie dinner to collect it on his behalf.

It's on such celebratory occasions that dieting determination seems to go to the wall. I had a glass of wine, sneaked a nibble at the potatoes and the tarte tatin. Guilt consumed me in the days after the event and I ate nothing but boiled or scrambled egg (skimmed milk and no more than a smear of the lightest oil), smoked salmon and the leanest of ham to make up for my indulgence. At that stage of the game, it wouldn't have worried me if I never saw another egg as long as I lived – just as I'd felt as a student.

As I prepared for the longest flight of my life to Auckland, I decided to enter the CONSOLIDATION phase of the Dukan diet, designed not necessarily to lose any more weight, but to keep off what I'd already lost. The first thing I planned to enjoy there was one slice of wholemeal toast with a little delicious New Zealand butter and the thinnest smear of jam. The thought of something crunchy between my teeth was just too exciting, as was the thought of having a good flat white with some skimmed milk. I had, in fact, got used to skimmed milk quickly, and now found fatty milk or cream too sickly.

It was perhaps a bit of a dangerous game to allow myself to salivate over things I wasn't really supposed to eat. The successful dieter is the person who devotes every minute of every day to wiping such delights from their mind for ever. I was simply visualizing something I would love and tasting it in my imagination.

I packed a bag of oatbran in case they didn't sell it in New Zealand, and looked forward to being able to eat fruit every day (not bananas), something light – maybe a small salad – for lunch, and for evening meals it would be pretty much what I'd got used to on the CRUISE phase – protein-only one day, and protein and veg the next – so lean meat, fish and, from what I'd heard about seafood Down Under, maybe the occasional crab or lobster.

The Sauvignon Blanc or Hawke's Bay Merlot, I thought, might be a bit of a challenge, especially as the Kiwis' excellent wine costs half as much as it does in the UK, but the thirty minutes of daily exercise I was expected to do on this phase would be easy. I wouldn't have my dogs to accompany me – they were going on their own little holiday to my friend Kate's – but there'd be lots of clambering around the rugby stadia and there's not much to do in New Zealand apart from walking the beaches, hiking the hills and swimming. I'd be fine. Or so I thought. It's amazing how you can fool yourself into thinking you're in control.

6

Shame and Self-loathing

For a while, then, I *was* fine. But during my three-week holiday in New Zealand I became unaccountably ravenous. Maybe I stepped away from the routine I'd established because I had slipped into holiday mood. What's more likely, I know now, is that my body had begun to rebel against the strict dieting I'd undergone. More of this will be explained in the science section in Chapter 8. We went out for dinner at a fabulous restaurant in Auckland and I scoffed the lot, pudding included, and drank a couple of glasses of wine. Then came fish and chips on the road with the boys and the alarming realization when I boarded the plane for the return home that the seatbelt fitted a little more snugly than it had on the outward journey.

By New Year, after a wonderful diet-free Christmas, I had regained 3 stone. It's amazing – and yet completely explicable – how quickly fat once lost piles back on again as you feed a new-found hunger. So, after only three months I was nearly 17 stone. By the time April came around I was back to the weight at which I'd started on Dukan – 19 stone – and I was drowning in the shame and self-loathing experienced by so many of us who have tried really hard and failed.

I suppose there was some comfort in knowing I was not

alone. That 95 per cent failure rate I'd discovered all those years ago still stands. Did I beat myself up about it? Of course I did. I was forced to go back to my clumpy, flat, boring shoes, because anything more elegant with some sort of heel was far too uncomfortable. I was only too aware of my resemblance to a chubby penguin as I waddled along the road. I knew I'd be perceived by friends, family and anyone who caught sight of me, having read my columns on my weight loss, as a failure who was LMF (Lacking in Moral Fibre).

But, again, always trying to look on the bright side, I went through the fantasy that I could be fat and happy – the jolly one, known for her sense of humour, well-stocked mind and acerbic tongue – and lay aside any more plans to be the slender, fit and active creature of my younger years. I would no longer deny myself my greatest pleasure – dinner out with the best of friends – and if I wanted a few chips or a chocolate fudge cake, I would have it. There would be no more diets. It was at this point that I pretty much gave up.

A meeting with the BBC's science guru Dr Michael Mosley prompted a rethink. I was interviewing him for the *Radio Times* about his latest TV programme, *The Truth About Exercise*. At that point he had not yet come up with his own diet plan, the 5:2. For the moment, he was concentrating on what he told me was a scientifically proven theory that one minute of high-intensity exercise three times a week, combined with a daily twenty-minute walk, is the only fitness regime the human body needs to remain healthy.

We talked, in passing, about my recent failure on the Dukan diet. Dukan had sold more than 11 million copies of his book worldwide, his company had registered a turnover of

£33 million and he'd had the best possible publicity when the Duchess of Cambridge and her mother, Carole Middleton, thanked him for helping them lose a few pounds in preparation for the royal wedding. But, even though some people had achieved success on this strictest of diets – and I suspect the successes had been enjoyed only by those who were looking to lose a few pounds for a special event, as the regime is so unsustainable – there had been rumblings of dissent for some time in France about Dukan's quick-fix formula of rapid weight loss. In 2011, his was voted the worst diet by the British Dietetic Association and a spokesman claimed, 'There is absolutely no solid science behind this at all. Cutting out food groups is not advisable.'

In the same year Dukan lost a libel case against a French nutritionist who told a magazine that his diet could cause serious health problems (though the court did not ultimately rule on the accusations from a scientific or health perspective), and a survey of 5,000 French people who had had success on the diet found 35 per cent had put the weight back on within a year and 80 per cent had put it back on within four years. It was, though, a serious allegation of malpractice that did the most serious damage to Dukan's reputation as a doctor.

In 2013, the French National Medical Board had censured him in the strongest terms for 'breaching ethical regulations' in 1971 in prescribing to a patient who wanted to lose a lot of weight a drug called Mediator, an amphetamine derivative believed to have killed some 1,800 people in France. The patient suffered heart-valve damage, thought to have been caused by the drug. Dukan, who had already voluntarily removed himself from the medical register when he retired the previous year, denied any wrongdoing and said he would appeal the decision, but it was a huge blow to a man who had long traded on being a respected medical practitioner.

Just as I'd felt after blowing the Atkins diet and all the other crazy attempts at weight loss I'd tried, I had an acute sense that I'd somehow been cheated. I'd been led down a garden path to misery by people who claimed medical expertise but, I suspected, had no real understanding of the complexity of the science behind weight gain and loss. I, and so many more of us, have placed trust time and again in the 'diet gurus' and they have let us down because it's so much more complicated than simply reducing energy in and increasing energy out.

Dr Mosley was hugely sympathetic to my acute sense of failure. He told me, 'We don't have enough long-term studies to show why some slimmers succeed while others don't, but we do know willpower is greatly overrated. Even people who have lost weight with a GP or dietician tend to put it all back on again. Of all the diets we examined scientifically, only Weight Watchers has a high success rate and seems to be quite sustainable.'

Now this was news to me, given everything I knew about the high Weight Watchers recidivism rate and a business model that seemingly relied on dieters coming back and paying to go on the same diet again once they'd regained the weight. I also had flashbacks to that brief period in the sixties when my mother and I had joined and she had obsessively measured every crumb she consumed. Could I really put myself through that again, along with the bossy group leader and humiliating weigh-in meetings portrayed in Kay Mellor's TV drama *Fat Friends*, which was broadcast from 2000 to 2005 and launched the career of a young James Corden?

Well, I had considered, albeit only in passing, having gastric band surgery, so joining Weight Watchers again felt a lot less drastic, especially if Michael Mosley portrayed it as a trusted, scientifically respected dietary regime. I decided it was worth a go. It costs £6.25 a week.

Weight Watchers had clearly come a long way since my mother and I dabbled in it in the 1960s. All the obsessive weighing and measuring appeared to have gone, and instead I was given a daily ProPoints allowance based on my height, weight and age. The system is designed so that each portion of food is assigned points for the type of calories it contains. A meal low in fat and high in protein would have a lower number of points; one with more fat would have higher points. My allowance was 36 and, on top of that number, everyone is given an extra 49 points that can be consumed across the week. The extras helped take the guilt out of the odd glass of wine – 4 points for a medium glass of red – and the occasional portion of fish and chips was OK (it carries 30 points). There are around two hundred foods that are worth 0 points, including eggs, skinless chicken breast, fish and seafood, legumes and most fruit and vegetables. Avocados, olives, mushy peas, parsnips, potatoes, sweet potatoes and yams have points that have to be tracked and recorded, and fruit juices and smoothies are high in points so best left out, as are fats and sugars.

After three or four weeks of sticking fervently to the 'healthy eating' regime, I had lost 6 pounds and convinced myself I was 100 per cent committed to the programme. I never quite summoned up the courage to attend the famous Weight Watchers meetings. I was definitely not ready to stand on the scales in front of other people, which is an ongoing WW practice but has always felt to me like public humiliation. Some people clearly gain a great deal of support and, in some cases, friendships from belonging to such a group. Maybe it's been my life as an independent only child that's made me reluctant to be clubbable in any way. Each to his or her own.

I did take up the offer of a leader, Julia, who was available on the phone to give me support, answer any questions and monitor my progress. We had our first meeting in a favourite Turkish restaurant and ordered the lunchtime mezze. She helped me work out that the meal would be 15 points as long as I ate only one very small piece of wholemeal bread and a tiny amount of the hummus.

Her advice on portion control was interesting. She assured me that spaghetti was allowed as long as you totted up and recorded the points against your weekly allowance. The portion for one person could be worked out by bunching the dried pasta together in the hand, holding it upright and, if it fitted on to a 5p piece it was the correct amount. It seemed surprisingly small, but it does, of course, swell up in the pot. A baked potato, which carries 3 points (no butter!), should be no bigger than a computer mouse and only one per meal is permitted.

As far as exercise was concerned, there was no pressure to get serious at the gym, but there were constant reminders that 'being active is vital for healthy weight loss'. The recommendation was to do a little bit more than before. I added an extra half-hour to the daily dog walk.

I also have to confess that I tried to get a little extra help. I had become a non-executive director of the Christie Hospital in Manchester where I'd been treated some six years before for breast cancer. The hospital has a complementary-therapies department where one of the therapists, Lynne, had developed a programme she called 'Emotional Eating and the Ethical Gastric Band'.

In for a penny, in for losing a few pounds, I attended dutifully week after week. Each time, she hypnotized me to believe I should eat only to satisfy my real hunger rather than my emotional hunger. I was given a CD to which I could listen at home and be reminded to eat only until I was full. I became acutely aware of Susie Orbach's advice to think of listening to my appetite, and only eating when I'm truly hungry and stopping when I'm full. I resigned myself to a slow rate of weight loss – Weight Watchers reckons 2 pounds a week is achievable – and for a few months managed to stay on track.

I quickly realized, though, that my fears that the sensual pleasure of a really relaxed, good meal with my family or friends would be lost were not misplaced. I was measuring things obsessively, from the size of any potato to whether the spaghetti would fit on the 5p piece. I was counting points, writing down every morsel I'd eaten and obsessively adding up the points consumed. Yes, I lost a few pounds, but my former obsession with comfort eating had turned into an obsession with uncomfortable eating.

Food had become a full-time job. And that early sense of feeling liberated from the need to gobble up everything on the plate, when I convinced myself it was OK to waste what I didn't want, soon began to dissipate. That old sense of feeling very hungry indeed began to kick in again. No amount of ethical-gastric-band talk could stop my body from telling my brain I was famished, and my brain from shouting, 'You're starving – go ahead, EAT!' The weight began to creep up again. Another failure.

I thought about giving Slimming World a try. A few friends

told me they'd found it really helpful, but when I examined the regime it didn't seem much different from Weight Watchers' sensible healthy-eating plan. And there would be meetings. Not for me.

Only one woman I've spoken to about this whole 'slimming' business who shares my sceptical, often cynical view of anything offered as a magical solution to the fat girl's nightmare is the freelance journalist Emma Burnell. Like me, she's an educated, intelligent woman who's now forty-four and, like me, has spent a significant amount of time and energy battling with her body's tendency to put on copious amounts of weight if she so much as looks at food. We arranged to meet after I read an article she'd written in the *Independent* on 4 July 2019, headlined 'I used to weigh 25 stone, but the responsibility for tackling the obesity crisis is yours as much as mine: Let's talk about what personal responsibility really means, and how you can make sure you're taking your own responsibilities seriously. Starting with not patronizing your friend who would "be so pretty if they lost weight".' That was a familiar story!

The article was responding to the Cancer Research UK advertising campaign that compared obesity to smoking. Emma was angry, just as I had been, at the criticism directed at the charity for what was described as 'fat shaming'. Emma too was keen to emphasize that we can't deny science, and science has shown that certain cancers are caused by obesity. As she wrote, 'Cancer Research UK is not fat shaming. Far from it: scientific truths are important and they can't be massaged to spare the feelings of those who are affected by them.'

She understood and shared the pain of those who know that every time the obesity debate is raised in public, no matter how sensitively, it will make life harder for those of us who are obese. The scientific facts are translated, as she said, through the lens of the media, social media and wider society, and it's the man or woman struggling with the shame of their own obesity who will be blamed for the cost to the NHS – said to be £6.1 billion a year and affecting 1 in 4 people – of their 'greed and laziness'. But losing weight, as she explained in her article, is a physical and emotional slog.

> It's difficult in a way that people who only want to drop a few pounds for the summer will never truly understand. But, because almost everyone has undertaken some form of weight control, everyone thinks they know how it's done. It is this that makes myths around 'personal responsibility' so prevalent. Many obese people know that the ultimate formula for weight loss is to eat less and get more exercise. But that's just not as easy as it seems. Being obese doesn't just change your body, it affects your mind. Knowing the facts and being able to act on them are very different things.

Like me, Emma had found her weight had yo-yoed as her circumstances and her consumption of food changed. She was, she told me, always considered overweight. As a teenager she had piled it on, rising to 20 stone before she was twenty years old. She had never really believed in dieting, and her fondness for what she calls 'bad food', mainly fried chicken with the skin on and chips, had generally been her downfall. She tried a vegetarian diet for a while and lost a couple of stone. She had a go with the 'fat-burning' drug XLS, which supposedly prevents the metabolizing of fat. She says it was horrible, caused a lot of loose stools and diarrhoea, and what came out was a rather alarming orange colour.

When we met, Emma had managed to reduce her weight

significantly. She had weighed 25 stone, was only 5 foot 2 and described her old life as one of constant pain. She couldn't walk 100 metres without her back causing her agony and she was very aware that people tended to think she was stupid. She self-medicated and that was generally through what she described as the endorphin rush of overeating unhealthy food.

In 2013, at her largest, she lost her job and her husband, felt a complete failure and decided it was time to do something radical about her size. She saw her GP and he referred her for surgery. She had a gastric sleeve operation and found she very quickly lost 8 stone. The surgery, she concluded, helped change her attitude to food and enabled her to develop better eating habits, particularly when it came to portion control. She began to have a greater understanding of the effects food had on her. Protein, she discovered, filled her up, but too many carbohydrates made her sleepy. Her portion size reduced considerably and she learned it was OK to leave food on her plate if she was too full to finish it. Like me, she'd come from a culture where cleaning your plate was expected.

Even after the surgery, now weighing 17 stone and having broken up with a boyfriend, some comfort eating began to creep in again, so she decided she needed more help to lose more weight and prevent any gain. She joined Slimming World, an organization that celebrated its fiftieth birthday in 2019. It was founded in 1969 by Margaret Miles-Bramwell, a Derbyshire secretary who weighed 20 stone. She had £200 with which to start her business and a rather clapped-out Austin van. Fifty-five women attended the first session in Mansfield, Nottinghamshire. Today, 7,300 groups meet weekly throughout the UK, following diet plans that are much the same as those worked out by Margaret at her kitchen table fifty years ago.

So, what appealed to the anti-diet Emma Burnell about Slimming World? The basic rules of the Slimming World plan are divided into three sections. First there's free food, of which you're told you can eat as much as you like. It includes lean meat, eggs, fish, pasta, potatoes, fruit and vegetables. The second section is measured healthy extras, involving small portions of milk (skimmed) and cheese for calcium, wholemeal bread for fibre, nuts and seeds.

Then there are the Syns. It's a term Emma hates, as no food really should be categorized as sinful, but she sticks to the plan and works out exactly how many Syns she can risk in a day. The number allowed ranges from five to fifteen per day depending on your weight-loss plan. 'Treats' such as avocados, chocolate and wine are counted as Syns – all the things, I guess, would fit into the 'naughty but nice' category! Emma has no trouble remembering their values. She's a fan of sweet chilli sauce. She tells me it has one Syn per tablespoon.

You really do have to watch what you eat on this programme. As one contributor to the Mumsnet website asked a friend who was disappointed at only having lost 1 pound in her first week: 'Are you sure you've been counting your Syns correctly? Try not to get too disheartened. One pound every week for a year adds up to 4 stone, so it's a step in the right direction! Have you counted every spoonful of sugar, every dash of milk in your coffee? Every teaspoon of anything synful needs to be a level teaspoon, not heaped. Little tiny things can add up to a lot of Syns if you're not careful.'

Emma admits that Slimming World membership feels a bit like a cult. She dutifully attends her local meeting every week and pays her £5. Apparently it becomes free once you hit your target weight, which you're asked to set for yourself when you join. Emma set 10½ stone as her goal and by sticking very carefully to the rules for two and a half years she's down to 13 stone. She now describes herself as no longer morbidly obese, but still obese and heading for being simply a bit overweight.

She doesn't deny it's extremely hard work to stick with the programme. It takes a great deal of time and emotional energy to make careful plans for everything you consume. Happily, she loves to cook, has a savoury rather than a sweet tooth and she's found Slimming World has genuinely altered her relationship with food, and she hopes it will last for life. Her shopping habits have changed and she's very careful to buy only the lowest-calorie fat sprays with which to spritz her pan lightly for any frying. No butter!

She plans her meals across the week, has a huge Slimming World book containing all the rules and owns a whole library of recipe books with the suitable meals she knows she enjoys carefully tagged. She also keeps a food diary. She has, she says, never been hungry and refuses to call the regime a diet. She was, at the outset, extremely cynical. She's now a complete advocate.

The weekly meetings, she says, are essential. She compares it with AA, Alcoholics Anonymous, where a group of people battling with an addiction – but in this case food – discuss the problems they have faced and encourage each other. She says she's made a lot of nice friends across the community. Yes, everyone is weighed, but she claims it's not done in a harsh or critical manner. It's all about sustainability and not trying to change yourself in a way that could never last. Keeping it up is the reason why anyone who's achieved their target weight is encouraged to remain part of their group, and the free membership they're given hopefully makes that easier. There is a Slimmer of the Week, awarded to the person who achieves the biggest loss that has been maintained. She was Miss Slinky on one occasion and was awarded a sash. At this point I think I grimaced. 'OK.' She smiled. 'Lots of people love it.'

It is such hard work, though, and Emma admits it's not for everyone. People drop in and drop out quite frequently and she told me about one woman who lost 3 stone, but then quickly gained 2 back. She was South Asian and found she was often invited to weddings that might last for three days and every rule in the slimmer's cookbook would be broken. Family and community pressures can make life very difficult for the person trying to change their relationship with food for life. Even Emma, who lives alone and, on the whole, has only her own diet to think about, admits she sometimes slips up. If she's invited to a party or a wedding she tries to restrict her intake, but doesn't deny herself. Just for a short while she goes Syn-free.

Emma has advice for friends of fat people on the question of personal responsibility. A lifetime change of behaviour, she says, needs a lifetime's worth of support and encouragement. The personal responsibility of those who are not obese but are concerned about the obesity crisis is to 'never fat shame people on TV in the smug belief you are doing the nation a service'. She goes on in her article:

It's not to loudly comment on strangers who are just trying to get through their day. And it's definitely not to put patronizing pressure on your friends.

No, that role is about being understanding when your friend wants to meet at the same restaurant again and again because she's worked out what she can have there that works for her. It's about changing your understanding of an obese person's relationship with food so you can support them in making better choices, not shame them into hiding their bad ones. It's about understanding the emotions that go along with eating for a large portion of the population – and doing your best not to trigger those when you wade into this debate. We all have a role to play in tackling the obesity crisis. As long as the sole burden falls on the fat, rather than looking at how societal attitudes are affecting them, the worse it will get.

I've quoted Emma extensively because it was such a relief to find someone who understood the problem in exactly the way I have come to understand it. And, frankly, I couldn't have put any of her observations or advice any better myself.

Nevertheless, I still haven't managed to persuade myself that Slimming World is for me. As Emma says, some people love it and it works for them. But I've looked at the recipes and, whilst I accept they are well ordered and contain most of the healthy food options I would choose for myself, I couldn't see myself cooking the sauce for my spag bol without olive oil, removing the fat from my lamb chops or bacon, or eating a banoffee pie with a base made of ten reduced-fat digestive biscuits with 60 grams of low-fat spread and a level tablespoon of sweetener in the mix of quark and Müller Light toffee yogurt. No butter, no sugar – frankly, I'd rather do without! And, as supportive and kind as Emma says her group manages to be, I still can't persuade myself that I could cope with the humiliation of the weekly weigh-in. Each, as I said earlier, to his or her own.

7

What Fat Feels Like

It takes an awful lot of courage to publish a book called *Happy Fat: Taking Up Space in a World That Wants to Shrink You* and allow, or maybe even encourage, the cover design to be a photograph of yourself with your more than ample belly exposed. In the image, the thirty-year-old Danish comedian Sofie Hagen grins with her eyes tightly closed, her hands grasp each side of her waistline and on her tummy are painted two pretty eyes, a tiny nose and, around her belly button, there are smiling, luscious red lips with a defined Cupid's bow. How I wish I, and so many of the women to whom I've spoken for this book, were brave enough and confident enough to say, 'Hi, I'm fat,' seemingly without a care in the world, and tell others to chuck out their scales, stop listening to people who ask about their health and learn to love their bodies.

Most impressively, Hagen relates an incident I know has happened to all of us, hence the title of this book, and she dealt with it in a way we would all have liked to, but didn't. Here's what she wrote:

> Two young men were walking towards me. When I passed them, one of them said, 'Fat cunt!' and the other one said, 'I wouldn't even fucking touch it.'

That has happened before, loads. My usual reaction is to ignore it. Ignore it and process it later. I'd love to say that my reaction is to take a brick from my bag . . . and scare the shit out of the pricks. But bricks are heavy and I'm not looking to fight (let's be honest: be beaten up by) anyone. So I usually lower my head and continue to walk, pretending it didn't happen. Later I will write an angry tweet or shout to my therapist. At this moment in time, though, something clicked. Or snapped. Or fractured. Or popped. And I started laughing. I tried to stop, but it was too late; the men had heard it. It was a deep, bellowing stomach-laugh . . .

It was funny that they were so transparent and that they assumed I couldn't see right through them. I felt in my gut that the opposite of cowering – of immense shame, of hiding and self-hating – is laughing, loudly.

And there we were:

Me: a fat person. A fat person who has spent upwards of eight years unlearning fat hate and learning self-love.

Them: just two random men. Two random men who have been bombarded with fatphobic adverts, TV shows, movies, stand-up comedy routines, news reports and history lessons. And whose default setting is to believe all of it.

If only I could have laughed. If only I could have learned to love my fat body. If only I hadn't been taught from child-hood that fat was ugly and somehow immoral. If only I hadn't opened the newspapers every day and found a zillion articles telling me obesity is a disease, obesity-related hospital admissions have risen in one year by 15 per cent, that obesity costs the NHS £6.1 billion a year, that here's a new diet to fix your fatness and here's another aristocrat/actress/Instagram influencer who's lost her baby weight in just one week. It's endless. It's pervasive. It's hurtful and humiliating. And I am absolutely not alone in finding it simply impossible to laugh off.

I've been honest about the way that fat makes me feel. But I'm just one person. Here are some of the conversations I've had with other fat women and some men who, like me, have longed to adopt the principles of body positivity and have singularly failed to do so. They are conversations conducted from a professional perspective, purely to inform my research. I have never spoken to anyone, friends or family, about my shame and self-loathing or about my size, nor have I ever opened a discussion with anyone else on a personal level about their own feelings concerning their size. It seems to be part of ourselves that we prefer to hide away under loose-fitting clothes and a carapace of indifference. I shall only use the first names of my interviewees. You see, shame hits us all and most of us don't want anyone to know our weaknesses. I remember Emma Burnell, who hasn't been afraid of her name being known, saying to me, 'I don't really trust anything or anyone not to hurt me!'

Jools

Jools is a professional woman of fifty-four, married to Paul, and has three children. She describes herself as a skinny child who, until the age of forty-two, after the birth of her third infant, weighed 9 stone 10 pounds. She's 5 foot 7. She put on a little weight in her mid-forties, but the serious gain began when she was forty-eight. She had pneumonia and was prescribed steroids. The effect, she says, was to make her so unbelievably hungry that she would get up in the middle of the night and eat half a loaf of bread. Her weight quickly rose to nearly 18 stone.

We had a long conversation, which is really something of a misnomer. For a good hour I barely managed to get in a word. Her anger and pain simply poured out of her. Perhaps some of these feelings and experiences are familiar to you.

I have this large lump of flesh. It's like an alien attached to me. And I've grown it myself. My face has kind of disappeared. I've got a lot of chins, hanging fat at the top of my arms and at the bottom of my ribs. I look pregnant. I feel like I'm carrying a seven-month pregnancy and it hangs down. I'm very careful of the way I dress. I wear big pants. Gone are the days of wearing anything sexy. I'm sad about that because you lose your sexuality. Well, I have done. It's the overhang. That's the thing I find difficult to dress for.

'Fat' is such a derogatory word. It's thrown at you. 'You're fat.' As I got fatter I became irrelevant in the workplace, my ideas were constantly dismissed. The men who're fat don't seem to suffer in the same way. It doesn't seem to be shameful for them. Sometimes people just say I'm bigger and think that makes it sound OK, but it's not OK. I am fat. I'm not happy to be fat. I don't like it. I've completely lost interest in clothes. Clothes used to be something I loved. I always made the effort to look nice. As I got bigger I became a bit of a hermit. I never went to the shopping centre where I might meet people I know. I was too embarrassed. Now to go shopping for clothes, which I used to love, is just practical and the aim is to just cover up how I look.

The number-one thing I think I feel is embarrassment and shame that I've allowed it to go so far, that I didn't deal with it when it started. I have friends who've had some success at Slimming World or Weight Watchers. One friend lost 7 stone at Slimming World and was actually Slimmer of the Year. She worked so hard at it, constantly obsessed with her diet, but I don't have much confidence in these clubs. They make a lot of money out of fat people. The science doesn't seem to support their methods. People go for decades, losing and gaining over and over. Professor Rachel Batterham at University College London's Centre for Obesity Research did a study on dieters. In women with a BMI over 35, only 1 in 340 had a chance of sustainable weight loss. It's a 95 per cent recidivism rate. They reach a goal weight and stop dieting. If the BMI is over 40, only 1 in 740 succeeds.

I do know that the only reason I got this fat is that I ate more and moved less, but it's a vicious circle. The fat makes me feel unwieldy and I can't move in the way I used to. My husband and I used to love walking in the Lakes. I can't do that now. We used to sail, but I can't do it any more because I can't move myself around the boat. It's frustrating because, as an intelligent human being, I know what I have to do, but for some reason or another there is something in my brain that won't let me do it. In all other aspects of my life I'm in complete control, but for this one I just can't crack it. There is some comfort in eating. Food provides a sense of pleasure, which, these days, I rarely get anywhere else.

I've got three children. We have a meal in the evening that is cooked from scratch. I don't ever have anything in the house like biscuits, crisps or any junk food. I eat good food, but my portion size is big. I eat far too much. Every single thing is an effort. It's horrible. In my family there's a lot of eye rolling – a 'Come on, Mum, get going. Don't be lazy.' And it is lazy because I don't want to do it. But I don't want not to do it in the conventional sense. I can't be arsed. I can't be bothered. I live in an absolutely stunning area, but I don't walk in it.

I have a slight advantage at the moment because a couple of weeks ago I had a cortisone injection in my knee. My daughter will often say, 'Do you want my arm, Mum?' I'm fifty-four years old, I shouldn't be taking someone's arm, but I do. I'm not obsessive about jumping on scales because it's so depressing. It's just a number at the end of the day, but it's an important number, directly related to the state of my health. I want that number to be lower. I'm hurtling towards type 2 diabetes. I have sleep apnoea, so my sleep is very poor. I'm so tired. I'm menopausal, but the GP was not very helpful except to prescribe anti-depressants, which helped, but apparently Mirtazapine is used as an appetite stimulant and seems to induce a particular longing for carbs. I found myself stopping for Cornish pasties at the bakery. I couldn't stop eating the wrong thing. My downfall was not sweets, it was savouries and bread.

As a result of the fat, I have osteoporosis and osteoarthritis. I have incontinence. I have high blood pressure. I've had a mini stroke. I don't want to die young, but, knowing all of this, I still can't lose weight. Sustainably. Walking, my breathing gets laboured, my lower back screams at me. I can't go for a walk on my own as I wouldn't be able to get up again if I fell. That would be a shame too far for me.

My relationship with my husband is very different from what it was. There's no doubt in my mind that he loves me to bits, but he doesn't fancy me and that's difficult. I do understand, though, because I don't fancy me. I don't want to take my clothes off in front of anybody else and certainly not in front of someone I used to have a fantastic sex life with. But I don't any more, and I haven't for a few years. I find it a very emotional thing to talk about. In fact, I never talk about it and we never talk about it, but we each understand it.

He's never going to turn round to me and say, 'I don't fancy you,' because you don't do that to people you love, but I don't even know if he wants to; all I know is that I don't want to because I don't love my body. I don't want to have sex with the body I've got. To have a good sex life you have to be fairly uninhibited and I'm about as inhibited as it's possible to be. He has a limited tolerance for the 'Woe is me, I'm so fat.' It's terrible.

After that I witnessed what was probably the first conversation Paul and Jools had had with each other about what had for so long been 'the elephant in the room' – not necessarily the kindest image to use in this particular case. First he talked about Jools rather than to her:

Paul: Her being fat has come very close to destroying our relationship. It's not about her becoming fat. It's the repercussions. The consequences of her becoming the way she is. I'm reluctant to say fat. I get defensive. She's my wife! To be brutally honest, the physical attraction's not there. I love her. I'm being as supportive as I can, right the way down the road. But the lack of self-esteem is the frightening thing about it. She's not dealing with it, which has led to her lashing out, so there's not a day goes by when there isn't a row. It's not about the weight, I think. It's about an attitude, it's about what's going on in her head.

Jools: The problem about the relationship, for me, is that the writing is on the wall. It doesn't always help to have it read out to you. So, whilst I can say it myself, it's always very hard to hear it from someone you love. It makes me upset to even talk about it.

Paul: I've never called you fat.

Jools: No, you've never called me fat, but it doesn't make it any less true. This is the first time we've ever talked about it. Ninety-five per cent of the time it is literally the elephant in the room.

Paul: We could handle things better, but not such an emotive subject.

Jools: The best thing for our relationship would be for me to be happier, without a doubt.

Paul: I want my wife back, but what I mean is, I want the wife back that's got a positive attitude, is happy, is confident in herself.

Jools: The 'fat and happy' idea is just not for everyone. It's most definitely not for me. But to make yourself feel better you've got to lose weight.

And there their short conversation came to a close, but I'm sure Jools' worries about her mobility and sense of dependence on her children are not unfamiliar to so many of us. I've certainly been anxious about needing to lean on my kids when really they should feel happy to lean on me. Nor does it surprise me that feeling unattractive and turning away from a partner you love because you feel embarrassed at the size you've become was a serious issue for Jools and Paul. You may want desperately to be loved and held, even feel you can still have an active sexual relationship, but it's hard when you think your bulk is getting in the way and you're afraid you might not be fancied any more.

Melissa

Melissa is forty-six, 5 feet 6½ inches tall and weighs 26 stone. She's an administrator in a university and describes herself as 'fat, black, a woman and disabled'. Her first answer to my question about how being fat felt to her was almost poetic, but terribly sad.

> I'm digging my grave with my spoon. I weigh myself every fortnight and I know I'm morbidly obese. I've tried and tried, but have consistently failed. People tell me I'm stupid because I am obviously not bright enough to understand what I'm doing to myself! As if!
>
> I know exactly what people think of me. They look at me and I can read the thoughts going through their heads on their faces: 'Lazy, slothful, ignorant, dirty.' When I attend meetings I tend to be ignored. People are very dismissive. They look down their noses at me and what

they're saying, without actually speaking, is, 'Look at you. You're unintelligent, lacking ability, unprofessional.' It really knocks your confidence, even though you know you're doing a perfectly good job.

I was always slightly bigger than the other girls at school, but not fat. I had that Afro-Caribbean 'bubble butt', which marked me out as a shapely fifteen- and sixteen-year-old in a predominantly white school. My mother is also fat. She sent me to Weight Watchers at one point. It didn't work. She went to Overeaters Anonymous. It hasn't worked for her, and her constant insecurities about her weight have definitely had an impact on me and my two sisters. She has a very complex relationship with food. She had a very messed-up relationship and became a divorced comfort-eater. She brought us three kids up by herself and she ate. My sisters are not as big as me, but we all have issues with our weight.

When I was a young teenager and a size 12, I was happy, but my mother wanted me to be smaller. She always looked askance at me whenever I ate. I never walked into my mother's house without her saying, 'That looks nice' or 'You look a bit bulky in the back.' Code for 'Good, you've lost a bit of weight' or 'Oh dear, you've gained weight.' I have no doubt family has a huge influence in this obesity problem. My grandmother was big, but I'm not sure if it's genetic or learned behaviour.

When I was at university I was very sociable and liked to eat and drink, but I think I underestimated how unhappy I was. My first significant relationship failed and I began to use my weight to rebuff advances. I have to say, though, there were not many overtures. They seemed to like skinny women best. I soon began to make jokes to myself about gaining weight. A favourite was 'You can't always find a shirt to fit you, but you can always find a cake that fits just fine.'

Friends weren't too judgemental, but as my weight crept up I began to notice people looking disapprovingly at my basket when I went to the supermarket, and I can't deny there was a lot of evidence there of considerable comfort eating. I love to cook and I think I became a feeder. It was a way of expressing 'I love you' to family and friends. Friends would always say how surprised they were at my weight gain because I never ate more than they did. I always gave them big portions and they saw me as generous, dishing out largesse, but taking care with my own portions. They didn't know I used to eat in secret.

As I grew older and began to work, I decided I needed to make a decision because I'd been drinking heavily to drown my sorrows. Fork or glass? I opted for the fork because I needed to be able to drive myself to work, and I couldn't do that if I continued to drink heavily. Food doesn't give you a hangover!

Increasingly, I find my relationships get more and more difficult. I really don't trust anyone who seems to show any interest in me. I haven't been out with anyone for ten years. The bigger I get, the range of people who show any interest in me diminishes, and the ones who do seem to me a bit dodgy. There are what I call 'chubby chasers' and 'fat fetishists', and generally I find any decent forty-seven-year-old bloke really doesn't want a forty-seven-year-old woman, regardless of her size. I don't think I'm considered an attractive woman. Pretty face, beautiful personality, but that's as far as it goes. I feel quite invisible, even though I'm so big.

I know my weight is having a terrible impact on my health. I suffer from osteoarthritis and fibromyalgia, and get very little exercise. I walk with a stick, and I know if I lost weight the impact on my joints would be so much easier. At work everyone leaves the office at lunchtime and goes for a stroll. I don't. There was swimming for a while, but I find it embarrassing to have to wear a huge swimsuit in front of everybody. I do endeavour, every Monday morning, to tell myself I will do it. I make myriad excuses.

I have a feeling I might have allowed myself to get to this size and stay this way as a form of weird rebellion. I have, to some extent, revelled in my weight and rather liked being invisible. I tried to go down the 'fat advocate' route, always ready to jump down the throat of anyone making jokes about fat people or discriminating against fat people, but I've had to admit that I've simply been lying to myself and lying to others. The only person this is all having an impact on is myself and I'm trying to stop telling myself lies. You think you're rewarding yourself with lovely food. You're not. You're punishing yourself.

Frankly, I'm bored with being fat. I never want to try to sit in a narrow chair in case I break it. And if I do sit down, I find it difficult to get up. I went for a holiday with some friends to Las Vegas and had to save up to fly business class, where I knew I'd get a bigger seat. I couldn't face economy. I'm so fat I'd be spilling over into the seat next to me. Even in business I had to have an extension seatbelt on the plane and then, once we arrived, I needed to hire a tricycle just to get around.

I have, of course, done lots of diets in the past. I did the awful cabbage soup one, Weight Watchers, Atkins and even saw an NHS dietician. With her, I began to feel resentful. What she expected of me was not my choice and I kept asking myself, 'Why should I conform?' Whichever diet I tried, I always lost some weight and then put it all back on, and some more.

I am, though, trying again. I'm doing the 5:2 diet for the second time. The first time I lost 3 stone and was so pleased with myself I went out and celebrated. Fatal! I've had hypnotherapy, and the message there was to think of choices. I mustn't think I'm on a diet, I'm just making more positive choices. I can't pretend the 5:2 is easy. It's taken me twenty years to gain all this weight. It will take a long time to lose it. I'm not going to go down the operation route as I'd be left with so much overlapping skin. I have to do this my own way. And I'm not listening to friends any more. So often they try to be kind and tell you you're not fat. We know they're lying and, if we want to deal with the problem, we have to tackle it ourselves.

It's so true that friends would never want to insult you by telling you you're too fat, although, in your mind, you know perfectly well they're thinking it. And then that sense that people must think you're stupid because you've let yourself get to such a size. There've been times, certainly, when I've thought, 'I know I'm clever and smart, but I suspect no one else sees it.'

Phoebe

There's no doubt the saddest conversation I had on this subject of what fat feels like was with Phoebe, who was only seventeen when we talked. She's 5 feet 11 inches tall and, at the time, weighed 17 stone. Her mother, Ali, joined us, not to chip in, but as a responsible adult there to take care of her daughter.

I'm not quite keen on the word 'fat'. It seems to have quite negative connotations, but that's what some people will label me as and I'm quite OK with that. That's their label, not mine. It can be quite rubbish at times, but then sometimes it can be quite lovely. Sometimes I love my body and sometimes I feel quite happy and then other days I think, 'Why do I have to have this fat on me?' And sometimes you wish you could just take it off. But then I think I'm coming to terms with it. It doesn't have to be such a bad sin. Except lots of people I talk to say fat is such a bad thing.

I always feel like an outcast. You say to yourself, 'Why have I let myself do this to my body?' People say stuff like, 'No one will ever love you,' but that's not true, especially when you start meeting new people. I think being bigger as a child meant I couldn't really be a child. I was obsessive about what I could wear to hide it. I can't even go swimming. Most children that age – around ten or eleven – go swimming. I loved swimming, but I got laughed at once in a swimming costume. I've never been swimming since.

I went through puberty very early and by the time I was thirteen or fourteen I really didn't like the way I looked. I was much taller than everybody else, and I had breasts and big thighs and rolls on my tummy. I suffered a lot of bullying when people would call me 'whale', 'gross' or 'fat'. I tried to reclaim the word 'fat', but it didn't make a difference. I did Brownies, Guides, gym and drama, trying to keep active. I loved drama because I like talking and acting, but I was concerned all the time that people weren't actually listening. They were just looking at my size.

I've really struggled with my mental health. In 2016 I suffered badly from depression and anxiety. In 2017 it got really bad and I stopped going to the gym. I had six admissions to hospital. Then, in April 2017, I said to myself, 'This has to stop.' I had treatment with CAMHS (Child and Adolescent Mental Health Services). I had counselling and dialectical behaviour therapy. It's a talking therapy based on cognitive behavioural therapy and helps you change behaviour that's unhelpful, but also tries to get you to accept who you are. I think it probably saved my life.

We talked a lot about weight and some of the reasons that may have caused me to be the way I am. I have polycystic ovary syndrome and I take medication, which may have contributed to my weight gain. I also have hypothyroidism and a slow metabolism, and have been very tired for years, with lots of broken periods. Mum has worried about me discussing calorie-controlled diets. I guess she knows dieting doesn't really work. I've never tried any diets, but I know my weight goes up when I get bullied at school. I have to learn not to compare myself with other people, keep controlling my portions and stick with a personal trainer, although my motivation is very poor. I know when I start to get anxious and depressed I eat junk food and comfort eat in secret. Most of the time I just feel guilty.

I found my conversation with Phoebe utterly heartbreaking. She is a child with a loving and attentive family who take great care to look after her in the best way they can. Her problems are many and absolutely not of her own doing. And, even if they were self-inflicted, what on earth do kids in school think they are doing bullying a girl about the way she looks to the point where she considers taking her own life? I'm not arguing that we should all become fat advocates, but fat shaming and discrimination simply has to stop.

Some months after my first contact with Jools, she got in touch to tell me she had made a difficult decision. She was convinced that her only option, if she was going to get her life and her marriage back, was bariatric surgery (now sometimes known as metabolic surgery). It involves reducing the size of the stomach by cutting away a part of it to create a narrow 'sleeve', or by making a surgical bypass. The intention in both cases is to reduce the stomach's size.

Gastric bands are a different process altogether, where the existing stomach is not reduced surgically, but a band is fixed around it to reduce its size and narrow the gap by which food enters it. The sleeve and bypass procedures cannot be reversed, but a band can be removed at a future date.

Jools had met a group of women who were all drastically overweight – some reaching anything from 24 to 30 stone – and they were trying to support each other by meeting regularly and discussing their progress. She had, she said, as a result, come to the conclusion that there should be far more help than currently exists on the NHS for people in their position, before they get to such a debilitating state.

Richard Welbourn, a consultant bariatric surgeon at Musgrove Park Hospital in Taunton, wrote recently in the *British Medical Journal* that Britain has the greatest number of obese people in Western Europe, but fewer of them receive gastric operations than in other European countries. He said we need to stop judging and start treating them. He believes that a safe, cost-effective therapy for a deadly disease such as type 2 diabetes – the major illness caused by obesity – should be made available for more than the 1 per cent who are offered it now. In fact, between 2012 and 2015 the number of gastric operations carried out on the NHS fell by 31 per cent from 8,794 to 6,032. Even as the numbers suffering from obesity rose significantly.

His conviction that all the clinical evidence points to the fact that, as a country, we should be performing more weight-loss surgery persuaded Jools to cast aside her family's concerns about it. She disregarded the 'don't take the easy way out' advice she was hearing from them and friends, and made the decision to go ahead with the operation, as some of the other members of her support group had done.

It was not easy to get started. She was classified as morbidly obese, with a BMI over the required 35, but the road to the operating theatre was long and arduous. First she was told by her GP that she must attend what's known as a Tier 3 weight management course, which might last for anything from six to twelve months. As access to a hospital where this kind of surgery is performed is something of a postcode lottery, the distance she might have to travel and the length of time the preparation would take would be dependent on her local clinical commissioning group.

She had to drive for two hours to reach her nearest bariatric centre. There were fifteen people in her group and at the first meeting 'someone', she said, explained food labelling. She felt she was patronized for forty minutes. The impression she received from the person leading the discussion was that the patients were all considered to be fat and therefore stupid.

There were three more such appointments between November and March. The second one was led by a dietician. Jools summed up her advice as, 'You must eat healthily and set yourselves a goal.' The members of the group were, apparently, appalled and insulted at being given the kind of advice you might give to children. As if these adults, who'd struggled with their weight for years, had no knowledge or experience of attempts at healthy eating.

The final group session, for which again she had travelled for two hours, involved a nurse explaining the different types of surgery that would be available. At that point the participants were told they had all completed Tier 3 and would now be put forward for surgery. The whole thing, said Jools, was a requirement, supposedly to prove that the attendees fulfilled the NHS criteria that patients should be put forward for surgery only if there was a clinical need. It was, she told me, a completely pointless exercise as it was apparent from the outset. The only thing that had been achieved in the Tier 3 exercise was that everyone in the group had put on even more weight. They'd tried to follow the dietician's advice but, as the time passed, they gained rather than lost. It's the case that dieting often makes you more hungry than ever and six months on a restrictive regime is a long time.

My encounter with Jools' support group came a couple of months after she had had her operation. It had not been, she said, a magic bullet, and she was nowhere near the slender

9½ stone she'd weighed before her weight began to go up, but she had lost 3 stone already and was beginning to feel like a different woman. She was having no trouble eating now she'd come through her post-op recovery period of consuming only liquids and puréed food, but she was finding she was eating mindfully and controlling her portions very carefully. It didn't feel like a diet, she said, and she was happily consuming everything from lentils to some meat, fish and vegetables, and she'd developed a liking for Skyr yogurts.

'If I'm hungry,' she explained, 'I eat something, and when I'm full, which is quite quickly, I stop. Why is this [surgery] not being encouraged? It's not done for cosmetic reasons, it's to save the life of someone who's morbidly obese. Why are there fewer bariatric operations this year than eight years ago?'

Why indeed? One can only assume cost and stigma, and the mistaken belief that we shouldn't be spending money on people who've brought their problems on themselves.

Half a dozen women were at the meeting of the support group on a gloriously sunny day in a town on the south coast. All were at different stages of their plans for recovery from the disease of dangerous obesity, and all had terribly sad stories to tell. Linda was fifty-seven years old and weighed 23 stone and 3¾ pounds. She knew precisely what the scales had told her that morning. Her problem had lasted a lifetime. As a child she'd been called a 'chunky monkey' and the advice to lose weight had been continuous. She had tried everything. A doctor had put her on a 600-calorie-a-day diet and she'd done her best. She'd lost 5 stone and had gone to a private cosmetic clinic for what she described as 'skin tightening and fat melting', for which she had paid a small fortune.

Not long after her weight loss she had been diagnosed with

type 1 diabetes and was treated with insulin and steroids. She had had to abandon the diet and, of course, had regained all the weight she'd lost. She was too fat to continue her job at an agricultural college and was becoming desperate about the state she was in. When she did manage to go out, young kids were cruel, making 'fat cow' remarks in the street. Her confidence was shot. A nurse specialist at her GP practice had suggested the possibility of surgery, but she was terrified of going ahead. Linda's last words to me that day were, 'I'm in a very dark place.'

Her words were echoed by Julia, Amelia, Jo, Tuula and Sarah, all of whom were in their forties and had struggled with eating disorders for years. Amelia had been bulimic during her teenage years and had spent a lifetime coping with depression and weight that constantly went up and down. It had now reached more than 24 stone. Her BMI of 40+ qualified her for surgery, but she was anxious about the fact that she would have to take part in her area's Tier 3 programme, which, in her case, would take place over six months. She found it upsetting that, despite her condition and her GP's recommendation, she was expected to 'tick boxes'.

Sarah, of a similar size, had spent a lifetime being reassured by a family who loved her and never wanted to upset her by telling her she was fat. They told her, 'Don't worry, love, you're just big-boned. Here, have a chocolate biscuit, it'll make you feel better.' Why, she wondered, would the people who cared for her, who could see the difficulties she had with food and fat, always seek to comfort her with cakes, sweets and chocolate? Like so many others, she had always been aware that her size made people assume she was stupid, and she said the most insulting thing that had ever been said to her was spoken by a nurse who made it clear she thought the problem was entirely Sarah's fault. The woman actually told her, 'Come on, it's up to you. Get some exercise. And when you're deciding what to eat, what would you prefer? A salad or a pork pie? The choice is yours.' 'If only,' sighed Sarah, 'it were that simple.' Her final words to me were, 'I know I need the surgery, but I need to get into the right state of mind. It's a big decision and it's not something to go into lightly.'

Sarah's story of a family that told her she was not fat but big-boned really resonated with me. It hadn't come from my mother, but my grandmother had often used the phrase in the hope of comforting me during my plump periods. And, of course, it's not uncommon for loving relatives to offer sweet things as a comfort.

Julia was also agonizing over the decision to go ahead with surgery. Her BMI of 40 also qualified her for a weight-loss op, but she was concerned about the requirement to attend four preparatory meetings over the course of a year before she would be accepted for the procedure on the NHS. As a busy woman, trying to work and earn a living, she was also anxious about the rule that, if she should miss any of those sessions for any reason or turn up late, she would be struck off the list. She had, some years previously, been diagnosed with type 2 diabetes and had managed to reverse it by following a strict diet but, of course, the weight had all been regained. She had not been tested again for the diabetes. She was very concerned about being seen as opting for a 'cosmetic' procedure and wasting the money of the NHS, but she knew she would not be able to sustain a diet without the operation. She was still trying to make up her mind.

Jo, at the age of forty-four, had risen to 25 stone after her marriage ended and she became the lone parent of three children. Her weight, which had been around 10 stone at the time of her divorce, had rocketed in only four years. She described turning first to alcohol to cope with the stress of her difficult new lifestyle. For two years she was alcohol-dependent and got through a litre of vodka every day.

She managed to bring the drinking under control in 2013 but found that, when she stopped, she became addicted to food instead. She never went to the shops, except to buy essentials, as she was too ashamed of her burgeoning size. Eventually, she was persuaded by her GP to join the NHS Tier programme in preparation for surgery. Her gastric bypass was performed in January 2018 and she quickly adjusted to the new way of eating small portions and never drinking alcohol or sugary, carbonated drinks. The weight began to fall away, to the delight of her now-teenage children. 'They say it feels like they've got their mum back,' she told me.

Nigel is not a member of the support group – I met him as the friend of a friend. He is a fifty-eight-year-old consultant in the NHS. He has always been a big man and was a semi-professional rugby player in his youth. It was when he stopped playing the game and had to work extremely long hours in the medical profession that he started to get fat. He continued to eat and drink every bit as heartily as he had before. He says he constantly asks himself why, with his professional knowledge, he didn't look after himself and wonders whether, if he could go back in time, with his awareness of the experiences he's suffered, he would take better care of his diet.

However, it was too late when his weight rose to 22 stone. His type 2 diabetes was out of control, he developed angina and had to have heart surgery, and his blood pressure was far too high. He became very scared, as the risks were piling up. With a BMI of 40, he was a candidate for surgery on the NHS, although his professional position didn't guarantee a fast-track.

He worked hard, in preparation for the gastric sleeve operation, to lose enough weight to shrink his liver and bring his blood pressure down. He had a terrible fear of the surgery and felt guilty because his need for going under the knife was caused, as he sees so often in his practice, by an unhealthy relationship with food. He walked a lot to improve his fitness for the surgery. 'I work in the system,' he said. 'I see all the complications. I know, if you get a complication, life expectancy falls off the cliff.'

The operation was a success initially. He lost 3 stone in the first two months and had begun to worry that the weight loss might never stop. Then it suddenly did taper off as his stomach started healing and he reintroduced more substantial food in smaller portions. However, he would add in what he described to me as 'some strange things'. They included the occasional nibbles, particularly crisps, and ice lollies and chocolate in the evenings. 'My enthusiasm for food is still there, but the appetite is not. It's a strange trap. I want to eat, but I can't find anything that will scratch the itch. I can't find the hit the old habit gave me. The joy and happiness, the old pleasure food gave me is gone. No matter what I shove in the mouth, that old pleasure is gone for ever.'

Five years on, no weight has been gained, but no more has been lost and Nigel is not a well man. The diabetes has returned and he's had urinary infections and bowel problems – he's concerned that his gut biome may have changed and made him more prone to bacterial infections. 'I feel a bit guilty,' he said. 'It's maybe my fault because I can't control myself. I am fat, but not as fat. The op works for those who make it work. It helps to reset the attitude to eating and it helps them make the necessary lifestyle changes. It's not a solution if you don't change your attitude to food.'

The only member of Jools' women's group who could be described as slim was Tuula. She's a forty-nine-year-old hairdresser who told me she had been big all her life. She had, on the whole, been quite confident about the way she looked, even though she had always been told to lose weight. And, of course, she had tried. Her biggest success had been with Weight Watchers when she lost 6 stone. But then she found she was constantly starving hungry. She reckoned her metabolism had been 'buggered up' (her term) by yo-yo dieting.

Her weight eventually rose to 25 stone and it was the difficulties she experienced in carrying out her job that finally persuaded her to make an appointment with her GP. At work, she had to stand all day in the salon and was beginning to find it so uncomfortable because she had difficulty moving around. Being upright was a terrible strain on her back, knees and ankles. Her clients were also not too keen on having their hair done by what she termed a 'beached whale' who was constantly sweating and quite often bursting into tears because she was so embarrassed.

Her GP revealed she had developed type 2 diabetes and referred her for surgery. Her husband hadn't wanted her to have it done, but she explained to him that the doctor had said that her life would be shortened without it. She had a long wait of a year and a bit before it was performed, but now, nearly two years after her operation, she was down to 10½ stone and her husband was very proud of her. She had eaten carefully, had no problems with hunger and, since Christmas – we met in the summer – she had found she could eat a wide range of foods in reasonable portions without gaining any weight.

She had no regrets, but was considering having cosmetic surgery to reduce the loose folds of skin, particularly at the tops of her legs. She was keen to wear shorts and thought she would have more confidence in her sexual relationship with her husband if there was less loose skin on her body.

She was, though, surprised at how angry she became at how differently she was treated now she was slender. She got really cross when men looked at her in an appreciative manner, hinting they now fancied her. She was very aware that she had been looked at in the past, but never in a seductive way. It had only been pity that she'd seen. She remembered that people had clearly thought she must be stupid because she was fat. Now men seemed so much more interested in what she had to say. 'Weird, isn't it?' she said. 'I've lost weight and grown a brain!'

It seems ridiculous, but I doubt that sense of anger is uncommon. Quite suddenly, as you lose the weight, people seem overtly to find you more attractive, more fun to be with and certainly brighter. I shouldn't feel cross when people say, 'You've lost weight, you look fabulous!' But I often do.

I so wish that people who deride the overweight and obese could meet and talk to the women and men who suffer so much heartbreak because of their size and the reactions to it that they receive. I'm thinking particularly of people like an old colleague of mine, the seventy-three-year-old, quite skinny broadcaster and journalist Michael Buerk, who wrote the most outrageously cruel *Radio Times* column in July 2019. The headline was 'Leave couch potatoes alone!' and claimed if people who are overweight were to live into their eighties and nineties, they would cost the NHS even more than the roughly £6.1 billion a year he asserted, correctly, that obesity and its complications cost now.

'How much,' he wrote, 'would he or she cost if, instead of keeling over with a heart attack at fifty-two, they live to a ripe, dementia-ridden old age, requiring decades of expensive care? The obese will die a decade earlier than the rest of us: see it as a self-sacrifice in the fight against demographic imbalance, overpopulation and climate change.' Naturally, he peppers his callous view of the question with all the usual pejoratives with which the obese and overweight are familiar. There were references to 'porky', 'guzzling' and 'being out-waddled'.

I would have thought it was a rather dangerous practice for a man who made his career out of television to be insulting, in a magazine read by people who like to watch television, the very 'couch potatoes' who might have watched him night after night when he broadcast the BBC news. And of course they would have read his words in the very magazine they buy to find out what they will watch on TV in any given week.

What is most dangerous about his view, which, of course, was picked up on and repeated in every newspaper and magazine across the land, is the conviction with which he promotes untruths. 'You'll lose weight if you eat less'; 'It's your fault'; 'It's your choice'; 'The truth is healthy food is cheaper than sugar-packed, fat-soaked convenience rubbish'; 'They're weak, not ill'. Most of the media seemed to go along with his assertions, although the modern scientific knowledge around obesity and thinness questions every one of them. What's more, he ignores the proven treatments such as the surgery we've been discussing that can help people lose weight, saving

lives and NHS funds. That his article was so widely dissem-
inated is proof positive that obesity is misunderstood and
openly shamed, even by people from whom you would expect
intelligence, thoughtfulness, knowledge and kindness.

I began this chapter with a story about one woman I consider
to be courageous, Sofie Hagen, the author of *Happy Fat*, and
I'll end it with another, the American model Tess Holliday,
who, in October 2018, appeared in a swimsuit on the cover of
Cosmopolitan. She's 5 feet 3 inches tall, is a UK size 26 and
weighs 300 pounds – that's just over 21 stone.

Tess is not what you expect to see on the cover of a fashion
magazine. She has a beautiful face and wonderful long red
hair, but her height, size, and her arms and legs (covered in
tattoos of the faces of her heroines Dolly Parton, Miss Piggy
and Mae West) are far from what's conventionally considered
ideal for a model or, indeed, ideal for any woman.

Tess spoke to the editor of *Cosmo*, Farrah Storr, about her
response when she received an Instagram message that
read, 'Fancy being on the cover of *Cosmo*?' Her immediate
reaction had been to forward it to her manager as she feared it
must be a joke. It wasn't, so Tess duly arrived in London and
prepared for the job of her life. On the morning of the fashion
shoot she woke up early, pulled back the bed covers, looked
down at her body and said out loud, although there was no
one to hear her, 'I'm a three-hundred-pound, five-foot-three,
tattooed mother-of-two . . . and I'm about to be on the cover
of *Cosmo*.' And then, she told Farrah, she wept.

As she prepared for the photographer to arrive, she explained
how she'd been 'trolling the haters last night'. One had com-
mented, 'You're so disgusting. F***, how many McDonald's

hamburgers do you eat a day?' Her response, sent at three in the morning on account of jet lag, read, 'Yeah, it's crazy, right? I just ate a tonne of Cheetos and I gained all this weight overnight. Weird, huh?' I guess she's learned that the only way to deal with such open hostility is to make light of it, but it must be painful when social media leaves you open to such consistent and cruel insults.

She explained to the magazine that her body had nothing to do with sitting around eating Cheetos all day long. When she hit puberty she had what she described as 'gigantic boobs and a butt. I was always different to everybody else. I have lived in a marginalized body almost my entire life.' She was, though, determined to bring her 'marginalized' voice into the mainstream, and she had the iron will to achieve it.

In 2013 she had been on the edge of success as a model. She had worked hard to get the occasional job modelling underwear and plus-size fashion, and was proud of her achievements in an industry in which everyone had told her she could never make it. She began to post photos of herself on her Tumblr account, along with short essays about how she was learning to love herself. She also wrote a memoir, which was part self-help guide, called *The Not So Subtle Art of Being a Fat Girl*. She wrote, 'I was not deliberately courting controversy, but it was clear that many people were not used to seeing photos of someone fat in their underwear. But for every ten people who loved it, there was someone who loathed it. The insults were always the same: "You're fat", "You're disgusting" or "You're promoting obesity". But my message was that everyone's journey with their body should be respected. There is too much pressure on people to look or be a certain way.'

Some weeks later, she found an online forum devoted to

discussing her body. Posters were saying she was too fat to be seen in a bikini and too big to wear stripes or show off her arms. She shot back on Instagram with a set of pictures and the words 'I want YOU to join me in wearing daring fashions and stop hiding your body because society tells you to. Break out those horizontal stripes and #effyourbeautystandards.'

As a result, the hashtag has been used millions of times as people posted images of men and women who do not conform to conventional beauty standards, and the fashion world woke up to the presence of a plus-size market that had often been overlooked. In 2015, Tess Holliday became the first model of her size to be signed up by a major modelling agency. By 2018, *Vogue* was asking, 'Will 2018 be the year of Tess Holliday?' But, behind the scenes, Tess was suffering postnatal depression following the birth of her second child and it brought with it a resurgence in thinking about the traumas she had faced as a child growing up in Mississippi.

Some of her earliest memories were of abuse. Her father had abused her mother constantly. Her mother left him, taking Tess with her when she was a small child, but subsequent relationships were a succession of inappropriate boyfriends who thought nothing of trying it on with a little girl. There was sexual abuse by a sporting coach when Tess was eight and she was raped at the age of twenty-two.

It was one of her mother's 'partners' who derailed her family life completely. In 1995, he shot Tess's mother in the head twice. She survived, but was left partially paralysed, and their rising medical costs meant they had to live in a trailer parked in her parents' garden. Her mother struggled to keep her children fed, often shopping in bakeries where everything was well past its sell-by date, or in one particular store where the goods had been damaged by tornadoes and hurricanes. It's as well to be reminded of how often abuse and poverty lead to eating disorders. There is clearly a psychological connection in all the cases I've gathered, although not all are the result of either sexual abuse or poverty. Depression brought on by stigma has a powerful influence on eating habits.

Tess met her husband, Nick, a graphic designer from Melbourne, on Tumblr. His first message to her was 'I love how you inspire women.' They dated long distance for three years before he decided to move to the States. He's the first man with whom she's had sex naked and, even though she's put on a lot of weight following her two pregnancies, he still insists she keeps the lights on in bed because 'You're too beautiful to have the lights off.' She says she now looks back and, although she doesn't wish she was smaller now, she wishes she had been able to love her body in her teens, when she was 120 pounds lighter. 'I'm at the heaviest I've ever been in my life now and it took me being the heaviest to finally love myself.'

I'm sure being loved has made a difference, as indeed must the success she's enjoyed as a model and having a husband with whom to share the pride in her career and the responses to her social-media messages, both good and bad. Being on the front cover of *Cosmopolitan* was, she reckons, the highlight of the years that have, on the whole, turned out very much for the better.

But, oh my! What a scandal that cover image caused. Piers Morgan, the presenter of *Good Morning Britain*, leaped in with shock and awe. His tweet in response to the *Cosmo* cover could not have been more damning. He reposted the picture and wrote, 'As Britain battles an ever-worsening obesity crisis, this is the new cover of *Cosmo*. Apparently we're supposed to view it as "a huge step forward for body positivity". What a load of old baloney. The cover is just as dangerous and misguided as celebrating size zero models.'

More than 16,000 of the twitterati liked his comment, one agreeing that *Cosmo* was wrong in 'glorifying morbidly obese people', whilst hundreds more criticized him for 'fat shaming'. Another accused Morgan of simply being biased against plus-size women because he'd also shown the picture of Tess on his Instagram account alongside his derogatory comments. One wrote, 'You aren't posting images of overly thin women on your IG saying how they promote an unattainable body image and can cause people to develop an eating disorder or orthorexia.' 'Orthorexia nervosa' is a term introduced in 1997 by a US physician, Steven Bratman, and describes an eating disorder characterized by an obsessive and excessive preoccupation with pursuing a healthy diet.

Tess hit back immediately and, unsurprisingly, the argument prompted a 'Twitter storm'. Tess typed, 'To everyone saying I'm a burden to the British health care system, I'm American, so you don't have to worry about my fat ass. Worry about what horrible people you are by whining about how me being on the cover of a glossy magazine impacts your small-minded life.'

Numerous supporters of the *Cosmo* cover argued online that Morgan had 'missed the point' of the cover, explaining, 'No, we are celebrating different body types and embracing who we are.' Another added, 'No matter what shape or size we are we should at least love ourselves. She loves her figure and I admire her. As someone who's had so many years of insecurities, it's amazing to see one of the many realistic bodies in *Cosmo*.'

So, Tess says her health is none of our business, and to some extent she's right. She should not be criticized for living in her body, which she's convinced is her natural state. I wish I could be as keen a fat activist as Tess, Sofie and so many more. I would never decry anyone for being fat. As I've made absolutely clear so many times in this book, I never want to hear anyone called 'fat cow' or 'fat' anything else in an insulting manner. But I hope these young women are not denying themselves the possibility of avoiding some of the damage that fat can do.

I, and so many of the people I've spoken to for this book, are of the older generations and we know what can happen with your health as a fat person as you age. Maybe I would have had breast cancer even if I'd been thinner. The four close friends with whom I shared the ghastly experience were all slim and fit, but all the medical evidence now points to there being serious risks associated with being fat.

The latest cancer research, published in the *International Journal of Epidemiology*, shows a distinct link between the genetic propensity for a high BMI and the risk of developing cancers. The chief executive of NHS England said of the evidence, 'The study shows obesity is a graver danger than previously thought. If we continue to pile on the pounds, we're heading for thousands more avoidable cancer deaths every year. Then let's not forget type 2 diabetes, generally caused by obesity, and the dangers of losing a limb or one's eye sight if it is left untreated.'

Maybe Tess has a point when she emphasizes her nationality. In the US healthcare system, where responsibility for paying for one's ill health is generally up to the individual and his or her own insurance company, a person's health is nobody else's business. I honestly don't believe that thinking can apply in a health system for which everybody pays, to which everyone is entitled to access and which is notoriously short of funds. No one who suffers from any health condition should be denied care and compassion, whether there is an element of self-inflicted damage or not, but we do all have a responsibility to at least think of the cost of our ill health – to ourselves, our families, and indeed the NHS – and do our best to avoid it. I applaud everyone who is doing their best to take good care of their weight and their health by whatever method suits them best, but I cannot applaud anyone who thinks it's funny or helpful, or just a point well made, to criticize anyone for their size – big, average or skinny. And please don't listen to those people, like the model Kate Moss, who say, 'Nothing tastes as good as skinny feels.' They're so wrong!

8

The Science and Psychology of Size

I am not a scientist. I got as far as a decent grade in GCE biology (a very long time ago –1966 to be exact). I am, though, a journalist, trained to analyse and explain even the most difficult of concepts and ideas. So, here goes! We're going to look at genes, evolution, hormones, environment, diet, stigma and fear of food, all through the lens of science. I have enjoyed very generous access to some of the finest scientific minds working in the field of understanding and dealing with obesity. The aim is to interpret what, it turns out, is a far from simple biological science to help us all understand why some people get fat and others don't; why diets work for some, but not for the majority; and what medical research has discovered in recent years that might help us deal with what can only be described as disordered eating.

Is It Your Genes?

I have always suspected that my two extremely obese late grandmothers handed down a genetic gift that seemed to bypass my mother and my father but made me a dead cert for a lifetime of grappling with my size. The genetic connection with obesity has now been confirmed by researchers on both sides of the Atlantic and, most recently, evidence of the huge role played by genes in the equation came as a result of work on anorexia nervosa, the very opposite direction to obesity on the road of disordered eating.

Interestingly, the eating disorder that causes boys and girls, men and women to become dangerously thin to a life-threatening extent has always been described as a disease. It seems to me, in the case of a dangerous disorder of this kind, whether your health is threatened by being too thin or too fat, the term 'disease' is entirely appropriate, so I'm puzzled that there has long been reluctance to define obesity in such a way.

A recent study, published in July 2019, emphasized the fact that anorexia nervosa is a serious and potentially fatal illness. The symptoms can include a dangerously low body weight, an intense fear of gaining weight, and a distorted body image. It affects 1–2 per cent of women and 0.2–0.4 per cent of men, and has the highest mortality rate of any psychiatric illness. The work on anorexia was a global study, led by researchers at King's College London and the University of North Carolina at Chapel Hill. For the first time, the conclusion suggested that anorexia nervosa, previously considered to be a psychiatric disease only, was also, partly, a metabolic disorder.

The research was described as a large-scale genome-wide association study, undertaken by more than a hundred academics worldwide. The researchers combined data collected by the Anorexia Nervosa Genetics Initiative and the Eating Disorders Working Group of the Psychiatric Genomes Consortium. The resulting data set included 16,992 cases of anorexia nervosa and 55,525 controls from seventeen countries across North America, Europe and Australasia. It identified eight genetic variants linked to the condition and the report underlined the fact that the genetic origins of the disease are both metabolic and psychiatric.

The key findings of the study were described thus:

1. The genetic basis of anorexia nervosa overlaps with metabolic (including glycaemic, or how different carbohydrates affect blood glucose levels), lipid (fats) and anthropometric (body measurement) traits, and the study shows this is independent of genetic effects that influence body mass index (BMI).
2. The genetic basis of anorexia nervosa overlaps with other psychiatric disorders such as obsessive compulsive disorder, depression, anxiety and schizophrenia.
3. Genetic factors associated with anorexia nervosa also influence physical activity, which could explain the tendency for people living with the disease to be highly active.

Dr Gerome Breen from the National Institute for Health Research Maudsley Biomedical Research Centre and the Institute of Psychiatry, Psychology and Neuroscience at King's College London was one of the leaders of the study. He said, 'Metabolic abnormalities seen in patients with anorexia nervosa are most often attributed to starvation, but our study shows metabolic differences may also contribute to the development of the disorder. Furthermore, our analyses indicate that the metabolic factors may play nearly or just as strong a role as purely psychiatric effects.'

Andrew Radford, chief executive of the eating disorder charity Beat, said, 'This is ground-breaking research that significantly increases our understanding of the genetic origins of this serious illness. We strongly encourage researchers to examine the results of this study and consider how it can contribute to the development of new treatments so we can end the pain and suffering of eating disorders.'

You may be wondering why, in a book about obesity, I have opened the chapter on the science of weight loss and weight gain with a discussion about anorexia. I was so struck by this new evidence, and the way it combines metabolic science and psychiatry, that I had to give it prominence. An awful lot of work has been done on the genetic influences on the metabolism affecting weight gain and loss in those who tend towards obesity, but I have been able to find very little on the psychiatric influences on weight gain.

The thing is, I know that my considerable weight gain came at a time when I was lonely and suffering frequently with depression and anxiety. My maternal grandmother struggled with what was then called manic depression and is now known as bipolar disorder. During her periods of being extremely low, she was often suicidal and underwent electroconvulsive therapy. My paternal grandmother was often depressed. Both, I believe, ate excessively because of a combination of their disordered mental states and their metabolisms. They both, unquestionably, used food for comfort. Neither drank alcohol, nor did they use smoking to occupy their hands and mouths. The men in the family enjoyed the occasional beer and smoked incessantly. The women found such habits unladylike and would invariably turn to a pack of biscuits, a bun, a bag of sweets or a bar of chocolate for their sensual pleasures in between ample breakfasts, lunches, teas and suppers.

At a time when the importance of mental health has risen up the political agenda, it is surely the moment when the dangerously thin and the dangerously fat should elicit sympathy for factors that are clearly beyond their control. And there must be more research into the psychological dimension of a person's tendency to overeat. Equally, if the anorexic's high degree of activity may have a genetic origin, is it possible that the overweight or obese person is not lazy, but genetically programmed to be averse to exercise?

Two of the specialists on whose work I've drawn – Dr Giles Yeo, the principal research associate at Cambridge University's Department of Clinical Biochemistry and author of *Gene Eating*, and Professor David Cummings, an endocrinologist at the University of Washington, Seattle – were both keen to emphasize the importance of the study of twins in understanding the role genes play in a person's weight.

Identical twins share exactly the same genes. Fraternal, or non-identical, twins share some genes, as you might with a sibling born before or after you, so there is not such a reliable comparison to be made in fraternal sets as in identical ones – the fraternal may well be as different in shape and size as any pair of siblings. The research on identical twins is what the two experts agree has provided unequivocal evidence that genes are vital to the understanding of the type of body size into which you might expect to grow.

Among identical twins who are raised in the same environment with the same influences, diet and drinking habits, more than 80 per cent will share the same body weight as adults. Of fraternal twins, also raised in the same environment by the same parents with a shared culture, only 20 per cent will have the same body weight as they grow.

Of course, that's not enough to prove that it's the genes that make the difference. Could it be the shared environment that makes them so similar? It was studies of identical twins who had been separated at birth and raised in completely different environments that confirmed it was genes and not environmental influences that determined the similarities in size and weight.

There are no accurate figures as to how many babies were separated in this way, but a 2018 documentary film, *Three Identical Strangers*, where male identical triplets found each other by chance at the age of nineteen, rather proved the point. They had been separated from their biological mother at birth and were rather callously sent to different families by an adoption agency supposedly worried that no adoptive parents would want to take on three baby boys. They were raised by completely dissimilar parents when it came to religion and socio-economic status, but when they finally came together they were physically identical and shared many tastes.

What they didn't know as they grew up was that they were part of a research programme conducted by the Austrian-born US child psychiatrist and psychoanalyst Peter Neubauer, who used identical siblings separated at birth to examine whether nature or nurture – genetics or environment – was most important in determining the kind of adult we become. Clearly, in this case, when it came to determining size and weight, nature triumphed. The first two triplets came together when they ended up in the same university environment and friends confused one for the other. The third of the three young men only came to light when his adoptive mother saw pictures of his two brothers in a magazine and noticed all three had identical, pudgy hands.

Their case demonstrates how many such children may have been separated without them ever knowing they had identical siblings. China's one-child policy is another case in point. *Twin Sisters*, a documentary by the Norwegian film-maker Mona Friis Bertheussen, tells the story of identical Chinese twin girls. The pair had been found abandoned in a cardboard box. Mia was adopted by a Californian couple and Alexandra by a couple from the north of Norway. Alexandra lived an outdoor life in a quiet village close to the Arctic Circle where there are periods when it never gets dark and others when it's never light. Mia was raised a Californian sunshine girl.

Their cultures, diets, education and the climates in which they were raised could not have been more different, but when they were brought together at the age of ten the similarities between them were uncanny, particularly their height and weight. As Dr Yeo writes in *Gene Eating*, 'Of course, the older the twins are when they are eventually reunited, the larger the influence of the environment and, consequently, the greater the variance in their weight. Time and time again, however, the power of genetics, even in the face of such environmental differences, is quite literally jaw-dropping.'

Evolution

There are certain ethnic groups that are more likely to become obese than others. The Pima Indians are Native Americans who live in the deserts of Arizona in the south-west of the United States. They are one of the heaviest peoples in the world. Nearly all are extremely obese and more than 50 per cent suffer from type 2 diabetes, a number that is five times higher than in the rest of the US, where, of course, obesity is not uncommon. The Pima are said to have been suffering from obesity for more than fifty years.

There is, though, another group of Pima who live in the Sierra Madre mountains of Mexico. They are the same race and they all began their lives in Arizona, but the Mexican Pima, who at some point in the past broke away from the others, have no tendency to obesity at all. The reason for the difference would appear to be only their environment. The Arizona Pima live the American way with all its excesses. The Sierra Madre Pima live exactly as their ancestors did. They are farmers with a subsistence diet and carry out daily hard physical labour.

A second example of how environment appears to play its part is in the different peoples of the Pacific Island nations of Polynesia. The small island of Nauru, for example, is one of the most obese countries in the world. Nearly 95 per cent of its inhabitants are overweight, of whom more than 45 per cent are obese. The Cook Islands, according to the World Health Organization, is the fattest place in the world, with more than 50 per cent of the population classed as obese. Samoa, Tonga and the Marshall Islands are not far behind.

As Dr Yeo points out, it's generally assumed that the obese Pima and the inhabitants of the Polynesian islands are as fat as they are because they exist in communities where it's culturally accepted that big is beautiful. Or maybe it's because of lifestyle. Are the Arizona Pima obese simply because they consume an American diet and the Polynesians because they exist on imported, highly processed food, do very little exercise and have poor healthcare? None of those glib theories tells the whole story. In fact, it's all about evolution and survival.

In both regions – the islands and Arizona – there had been millennia of adaptations to fluctuations in the availability of food. For the Pima, the landscape was harsh, and the islanders were isolated geographically. In both cases there was an abrupt alteration in circumstances that led to a change in the type of food available and reduced the necessity for hard physical labour to obtain nutrition from the products of farming or fishing. For both populations, life had been extremely harsh and they had lived through periods of feast and famine. What Dr Yeo describes as a 'genetic premium' would have been created in those individuals who were best able to endure periods when there was a high risk of starvation.

The individuals who were better able to eat more and store the fat during times of plenty, and were also able to conserve energy during shortages, were more likely to survive the hard times. Those genes were likely to be passed on to their children and you have an evolutionary process that could, I suppose, be defined as 'survival of the fattest'.

The Arizona Pima's supply of food was threatened in the 1920s when the US government stopped the flow of the Gila River upon which the Pima had depended. A dam was built upstream of their native lands to create an irrigation project that was of no use to them. Their water supply was lost and they were no longer able to irrigate their land or grow their own food. The Pima became reliant on government food handouts, which were processed and higher in sugar and refined flour than the food to which they were used. Their evolved genes, which gave them healthy appetites and the ability to retain fat, led to a rapid increase in obesity levels.

The Polynesians, used to living in fishing communities and having formed their island states as a result of arduous sea journeys across the vast Pacific Ocean, had developed a similar gene structure to that of the Pima, where being big meant survival. In their case too, it was Western influence that changed their way of life. The Americans and the British set up airbases in the region during the Second World War. Mining opportunities on some of the islands were discovered and the islanders began to be affected by globalization, which included the importation of the Western diet. The food was cheap and dense in calories. The inevitable happened.

The question remains – why are all of us, who so often eat the same foods as the ones to which these communities turned, not also universally grossly obese? It's believed that the vast majority of those of us whose ancestors evolved on continental plains were able to move elsewhere if they encountered famine and did not need to develop the genes that would enable survival. But, as Yeo says of the survival genes, 'While those genes were advantageous and enabled survival in a feast–famine environment, they have become deadly in today's feast–feast environment.' I can only assume that somewhere in my dim and very distant past were ancestors who had a very rough time when it came to finding their food.

Nor am I alone. The average weight and height of our twenty-first-century Western population has increased because we all have more food and, given the forms of transport available to us and the reduction in manual labour, we all move around less. Those of us who have inherited the survival genetic variation have become more obese than others.

Professor Cummings, in our conversation about the fat gene and the skinny gene, told me that common obesity can be the result of slight variations in hundreds of genes that contribute to our energy levels and our appetite. As we inherit our genes from both our parents, it's perfectly possible to have a sibling who inherits the skinny gene whilst you have the fat one.

In his own family, he told me, there was a real problem for his parents. They would sit down to dinner as a family and his very skinny father would eat one hamburger and be perfectly satisfied. His mother would eat three. His father would remonstrate with her at virtually every meal. Why did she have to eat so much more than everyone else when she was becoming so obese? She would simply reply that she was still hungry. It was a source of constant upset for her, and her son's fascination with the problem led him to train as a doctor and make the study of endocrinology his life's work.

Evidently, some of us are made to feel more hungry than others, and it's easy not to eat when you don't feel hungry. It's also hard to stop if you have a greater-than-average appetite, but that's what we fatties experience all the time. It's a constant struggle. As Professor Cummings says, 'Body weight is primarily genetic. We should define [obesity] as a genetic disease, no different from sickle cell anaemia or haemophilia. Disease is an entirely appropriate name for it. The obese are not greedy, lazy or immoral. They are fighting their biology.'

It's interesting that Dr Yeo is often asked whether his research on genes is not simply providing obese people with an excuse for getting fat. He points out that it's a question that's only asked about the genetics of what might be described as a behaviour – eating too much. He doubts whether he would be asked the same question if he were studying the genetics of heart disease or arthritis or Alzheimer's or Parkinson's. Clearly, his work would not be giving people suffering from those diseases an excuse for their illness. He says that he and everyone working in the field of obesity genetics is trying to understand the biology underlying the problem. It's only by understanding the science of obesity that we can begin to fix it.

Is It Yer 'Ormones, Love?

I remember years ago we feminists used to get so cross at that question, knowing it was being used as an implied criticism of any erratic or irritable behaviour that would inevitably be put down to PMT. It generally had nothing to do with menstruation or any other aspect of female biology – we might just be annoyed or confused, as any man or woman might be, and we would respond with fury, 'No, I am not ruled by my hormones.' We might, in certain circumstances, have been wrong, but the science applies equally to men and women.

There are many different hormones circulating in the human body and they're best described as chemicals made by specialist cells, usually within an endocrine gland. They are released into the bloodstream to send a message to another part of the body, forming an internal communication system between cells located in different areas. There may be communication between one endocrine gland and another, or between an endocrine gland and a target organ – for example, when the pancreas releases insulin, which causes muscle and fat cells to take up glucose from the bloodstream. The complex interplay between the glands, hormones and organs is known as the endocrine system and affects a huge range of activities, including growth, puberty, fertility, metabolism and appetite. It's the two main hormones affecting appetite that concern us here: leptin and ghrelin.

Scientifically naive as I have long been, during my obesity research I found what I considered to be a staggering fact concerning the human brain. According to Professor Tim Spector, the genetic epidemiologist from King's College London, the brain uses 20–25 per cent of our daily energy resources, which

suggests that, as the command-and-control centre of our existence, it is the busiest, most active part of our body. It plays a
crucial role in controlling our hunger and weight.

I'm interested – and so should we all be – in why diets so
often fail. Our genes, hormones and brain work together, and
when we lose a lot of weight the alarm signals ring loudly. 'She's
starving. Quick. Make her hungry. Let her eat as much as she
likes. Don't let her feel full.' It's why so many of us can do so well,
throwing ourselves at weight-loss diets and hiring a personal
trainer to slim down, post pictures of our new selves on Instagram as some public figures like to do, and receive widespread
praise in the tabloids for our amazing self-control. Maybe we'll
continue to succeed by employing an iron will, but at some
point, the hunger hormones will kick in, our bodies will think
we're starving and we'll either continue the painful struggle
against our appetites or we'll become members of the 95 per
cent who regain all the weight – and more – after dieting.

It's a hormone called leptin that plays the biggest role in
this process. Its function was first discovered in 1949 at the
Jackson Laboratory in Maine in the US, when a researcher
noticed two unusually fat mice. One was named Obese, the
other Diabetes. Both had type 2 diabetes, both were identically
huge, resembling grey tennis balls, and they both ate like little
pigs. Experiments were carried out, which to me, an animal
lover, sound positively barbaric. Each was stitched to a normal-
size mouse and then to the other to see what happened when
they shared their circulatory systems. Such experiments, mercifully, are no longer carried out.

Early results led to the discovery that there was some hith-
erto unknown substance in the mice's systems that influenced
their hunger and overeating. Further research carried out in

subsequent years, as genetic work became more sophisticated, led to the laboratory of Jeffrey Friedman at the Rockefeller University in New York reporting in 1994 that the obese mouse had a gene mutation in a hormone named leptin – from the Greek *leptos*, meaning thin. Leptin, it was found, is made in fat cells and travels to the bloodstream, where it circulates inhibiting appetite. When leptin was injected into the obese mouse, the animal stopped eating and shrank in size. It was the first hard evidence of the existence of a hormone system that could regulate food intake and showed the tendency to thinness or obesity was far more complicated than simply being about greed or willpower.

Experiments carried out in subsequent years on alarmingly obese little children found that injecting them with leptin reduced their feelings of hunger considerably and they went down to an average weight for a child of their age. The diet and pharmacological industries became terribly excited, convinced they had found the cure for obesity. They were wrong. Lots of people went on to be injected with leptin to no effect. Researchers then realized that, as long as you had a system in which leptin functioned as it should, an extra injection made no difference. The children who appeared to have been helped by the treatment had a complex fault that meant they had no leptin in their systems at all before they were injected.

It's now understood, as a result of work at Harvard University, that leptin only does its job when there is not enough of it circulating in the body. The hormone's role is to tell the brain how much fat you are carrying. Fat is your energy store, so how much fat you have is related to how long you would last without eating any food. If you have plenty of fat, generally you have plenty of leptin circulating, which tells your brain all is well. As you diet and lose weight and fat, the level of leptin falls. The brain then receives the message that your fat stores are dwindling and you're going to starve!

This is what happens to so many of us when we're feeling proud of ourselves for having lost so much weight. The fall in leptin turns on the starvation response, which makes the brain instruct us to find food and eat. Meanwhile, the brain orders the body to shut down unnecessary and metabolically expensive functions in order to preserve nutrients and energy to enable us to find food, gain weight and produce more leptin in the regained fat. The normal functioning of our reproductive and immune systems is immediately put at risk until the brain's fear of dying from starvation is allayed.

In his book, *Gene Eating*, Dr Yeo illustrates this effect with the story of a conversation he had with a London cabbie on a wet winter's day in the capital. He'd explained to the driver that he was in a hurry to get to King's Cross to catch a train back to Cambridge. The cabbie asked him what he did in Cambridge. Giles told him he studied food intake and obesity. The conversation went as follows:

'Yeah, you know, I just started a f***ing diet two weeks ago. I've got two f***ing stone to lose.'

'What kind of diet are you trying?'

'F***ing Slimming World,' says the disgruntled cabbie.

'Oh, is that like Weight Watchers?'

'Slimming World, f***ing Weight Watchers, they're all the f***ing same. While you're weighing in weekly, you stay motivated to lose the f***ing weight. You don't wanna feel like a f***ing loser,' says the cabbie, getting into his stride. 'The moment you stop, all the f***ing weight comes back on. That's the problem with all these f***ing diets . . . they only work when you're f***ing on them.'

Giles winds up the story, 'I nearly killed myself f***ing laughing. But he was, of course, entirely correct.'

Ghrelin is the second hormone that affects the appetite. It's produced and released mainly in the stomach, with small amounts also sent out by the small intestine, pancreas and brain. It has a number of functions, but it's known as 'the hunger hormone' because it stimulates appetite, increases our intake of food and plays a role in the promotion of the storage of fat. In experiments where it has been administered to humans, it can increase a person's food intake by up to 30 per cent. It acts in the brain on the hypothalamus, an area that is crucial in the control of appetite. It also acts on the amygdala, which is where the brain's reward system is based. It's where, on the left side, we experience joy, euphoria and pleasure. The right amygdala is where we process fear. I guess for those of us who fear that food will make us fat, it's having as much influence as it has on those of us who love to eat for the pleasure it gives us.

Ghrelin levels are primarily regulated by the intake of food. Levels of ghrelin in the blood rise just before eating and when fasting, but the timing of the rise of the hormone is generally affected by a normal meal routine. So ghrelin is thought to play a major role in the mealtime hunger pangs. Eating reduces the concentration of ghrelin, and different nutrients slow down ghrelin release to varying degrees. Carbohydrates and proteins restrict its production and release to a greater degree than fats.

Ghrelin levels increase after dieting, which, combined with the impact of the fall in leptin levels as a result of the loss of fat, contributes to the explanation of why dieting rarely results in long-term loss of weight. Curiously, ghrelin levels are usually lower in people with a higher body weight than in those who are slim, which suggests elevated ghrelin levels are not a cause of obesity, although, according to the Society for Endocrinology, there is a suggestion that obese people are more sensitive than others to the hormone, but more research is needed to confirm this theory.

Ghrelin plays an important role in the genetic disease Prader–Willi syndrome, where individuals affected are severely obese, experience constant and extreme hunger, and have learning difficulties. They have very high amounts of ghrelin circulating in their system and it's assumed that those levels, which are already high before the development of obesity, contribute greatly to increased appetite and weight gain.

So, yes, love, yer 'ormones play a significant role.

Metabolism

You often hear people blame their weight gain on their metabolism. They've cut down on calories and they're walking every day, but they're not losing weight. Could it be their metabolism is slow? Metabolism describes all the biological processes we've been discussing, and more, which go on all the time inside you to keep you alive and keep everything functioning. The minimum amount of energy your body needs to carry out these processes is called the basal metabolic rate (BMR) and it accounts for 40–70 per cent of your body's daily energy requirements, depending on your age and lifestyle. And yes, some people have a faster metabolism than others.

Body size, age, gender and genes all have a role to play in the speed of your metabolism. Muscle cells need more energy to operate than fat cells, so people with a greater muscle mass than fat tend to have a faster metabolism, but then, as we get older, we tend to gain fat and lose muscle, so our metabolism generally slows down as we age. Men tend to have faster metabolisms than women because they have a greater muscle mass, heavier bones and less body fat than women, and genes play an important role in determining muscle and bone structures (back to my mother and the 'What a pity you inherited Daddy's build and not mine!').

There appears to be little evidence that a slow metabolism makes weight loss difficult. Surprisingly, overweight people tend to have a faster metabolism than those who are slim, because larger bodies require more energy to carry out the basic metabolic functions. Dr Yeo uses a motoring analogy to explain this apparent anomaly. He compares a Mini Cooper with a Range Rover: 'While a Mini might seem to be very agile compared to the larger vehicle, it clearly has a far lower fuel consumption than a Range Rover. The larger engine and bigger mass to move about demands more fuel. The same is true for humans (and, in fact, all living creatures).'

It's generally accepted that weight is gained by eating more than your body needs, but there is evidence that metabolism slows as a result of crash or faddy diets. With some diets, the body is forced to break down muscle to use for energy, and the lower your muscle mass the slower your metabolism. It's another answer to why it's so easy for the body to put fat back on when you come off a diet.

Environment

In August 2018, the *Guardian* columnist George Monbiot asked a very important question. The headline read, 'We're in a new age of obesity. How did it happen? You'd be surprised.' He had seen a photograph in the newspaper of Brighton Beach in 1976 and could hardly believe it was taken in the same country he inhabits today, nearly fifty years on – an incredibly short period in evolutionary terms. Almost everyone in the photo was slim and he said it felt as if it were showing an alien race. How, he wondered, have we grown so fat so fast?

Monbiot was unable to find any consistent obesity data in the UK before 1988, at which point the number of obese people had begun to rise sharply. In the United States the figures go back much further and curiously, by chance, the moment when people began to get fatter in the US was around the time that photograph was taken, and the trend has continued ever since.

When he posted his thoughts on social media he received lots of responses. The obvious explanation, according to the majority, was that we were eating more than in the seventies when, several suggested, food in Britain was pretty disgusting and expensive. Fish and chips were never hard to find, but had pretty rigid opening times around dinner and tea, there were far fewer fast-food outlets and the shops shut earlier so, if you hadn't shopped for the day, you made do or went hungry.

Surprisingly, this assumption was wrong. According to figures from the government, we were eating more in 1976. The average daily calorie consumption in 2018 was 2,130, which included sweets and alcohol. In 1976 we consumed 2,280

FAT COW, FAT CHANCE

calories, excluding sweets and alcohol, and 2,590 when they were included. That's a significant difference. Other respondents on social media insisted that the cause must be the decline in manual labour. It seems to make sense, but the data doesn't support it. A 2017 report in the *International Journal of Surgery* said that 'adults working in unskilled manual professions are over four times more likely to be classified as morbidly obese compared with those in professional employment'.

Lack of exercise was put forward as an explanation by some people, saying that because we drive rather than walk or cycle, order our shopping online and spend our lives in front of one screen or another, we are much less active than we used to be. Not so, according to a long-term study at Plymouth University that shows the level of physical activity among children is much the same now as it was fifty years ago. A paper in the *International Journal of Epidemiology* found that, corrected for body size, there is no difference between the number of calories burned by people in rich countries and those in poor ones where subsistence agriculture and hard physical work is the norm. (There could, of course, be an element here of the growing popularity of cycling, gyms and running in the richer countries becoming a substitute for hard physical labour – my theory!)

The same paper proposes that there is no relationship between physical activity levels and weight gain. Numerous other studies suggest that exercise, while crucial to other aspects of good health such as mobility and cardiovascular function, is far less important than diet in regulating our weight. Some studies suggest it plays no role at all as the more we exercise, the hungrier we become and the more we eat. We all know the stories of people who end a long walk, a swim or an hour in the gym with a hot chocolate and a bun, or a pie and a pint, as a treat!

Some people suggested less well-known possibilities – adenovirus 36 infection (described as a human 'common cold' virus, easily caught from someone who is coughing or sneezing, and found to cause obesity), antibiotic use in childhood, and endocrine-disrupting chemicals that can be found in pesticides, metals, additives in foods and personal-care products – may play a role in the development of certain cancers, damage to the immune system, and obesity. Monbiot acknowledges there is some evidence suggesting they might all play a role and could explain some of the variation in the weight gained by different people on similar diets, but none appeared powerful enough to explain the general trend.

The light, he says, begins to dawn when you look at those nutrition figures in more detail. Yes, we ate more in 1976, but differently. Today we buy half as many eggs, but a third more breakfast cereals. We buy half the amount of potatoes, but three times the number of crisps. Direct purchases of sugar have declined sharply, but the sugar we consume in drinks and confectionery is likely to have rocketed.

My mother never bought fizzy, sugary drinks except once a week when we had a bottle of pop to share as a treat. She never bought fruit juice. We ate oranges as fruit for the vitamin C and generally only one at a time. It takes up to six oranges to make a glass of juice and that can contain as much sugar as a can of Coke. Best to eat fruit, rather than drink it. As Monbiot says, the opportunities to load our food with sugar have boomed.

The journalist Jacques Peretti, in his series of three films for BBC2 called *The Men Who Made Us Fat*, first pointed the finger at Earl Butz, the US Secretary of Agriculture in the 1970s, who encouraged US farmers to grow huge quantities of corn. The surplus was turned into high-fructose corn syrup (HFCS), which began to be used as a cheaper alternative to sugar in foodstuffs, from ketchup and pizza sauce to cakes, biscuits and soft drinks. By 1984, both Coca-Cola and Pepsi had replaced sugar with HFCS in their drinks.

The drinks got bigger too, to the extent it was not unusual to see people in the cinema or at the football ground carrying the equivalent of a bucketful of sweet, fizzy liquid, but HFCS, it turned out, was even worse for us than sugar. It was discovered that fructose can suppress leptin, the hormone that carries the message to the brain that you're full and should stop eating or drinking. The food industry was promoting foods and drinks that were bypassing our natural appetite-control mechanisms.

In his *Guardian* article, drawing on Peretti's investigative journalism, Monbiot describes how food companies are investing heavily in packaging and promoting their products to

> break down what remains of our defences, including through the use of subliminal scents. They employ food scientists and psychologists to trick us into eating more than we need, while their advertisers use the latest findings in neuroscience to overcome our resistance. They hire biddable scientists and think tanks to confuse us about the causes of obesity. Above all, just as the tobacco companies did with smoking, they promote the idea that weight is a question of 'personal responsibility'. After spending billions on overriding our willpower, they blame us for failing to exercise it.

It seems the personal-responsibility propaganda has worked brilliantly. The responses on social media to the beach photo taken in 1976 and the debate about why so many of us have become fat echoed the view that 'there are no excuses. Take responsibility for your own lives, people.' 'No one force feeds you junk food, it's personal choice.' 'It's everyone's right to be lazy and fat because there is a sense of entitlement about getting fixed.' As Monbiot writes, 'We delight in blaming victims.'

He also points to the fact that a paper in the medical journal *The Lancet* explained that 90 per cent of policymakers believe that 'personal motivation is a strong or very strong influence on the rise of obesity'. That suggests the politicians who may have the power to influence the food industry do not take into account the mounting evidence of what is really contributing to the obesity crisis, which has seen 64 per cent of English people become overweight or obese. We hear there's pressure to reduce the amount of sugar in soft drinks and raise the price of such items, then another politician appears dismissive of the need to exercise such control. Confusion reigns!

Monbiot suggests that what he calls 'obesophobia' may be a form of snobbery, because in most rich nations obesity rates are much higher at the bottom of the socio-economic scale. The scientific literature shows how lower spending power, stress, and anxiety and depression associated with low social status make people more vulnerable to bad diets. He ends his article with a plea: 'Just as jobless people are blamed for structural unemployment, and indebted people are blamed for impossible housing costs, fat people are blamed for a societal problem. But, yes, willpower needs to be exercised – by governments. Yes, we need personal responsibility – on the part of policymakers.

And, yes, control needs to be exerted – over those who have discovered our weaknesses and ruthlessly exploit them.'

My conversation with Francesco Rubino, Professor of Metabolic Surgery at King's College London and a consultant surgeon at King's College Hospital, and the man who you'll find in the next chapter was to become my 'fat chance', confirmed such anxieties about the role of the food industry in causing the obesity epidemic, but he was less damning than Peretti and Monbiot in his analysis of motives. The use of chemicals to preserve food for longer, or materials to make it taste better and cost less to buy, is not a deliberate policy to cause harm, he argues, but a government and an industry in the process of trying to help to cure poor nourishment. His concern now is the lack of scientific evidence available to policy-makers on which they might base their decisions. There is, he told me, as yet no clear scientific evidence that sugar causes obesity. (He does not include in this high-fructose corn syrup, which is thoroughly, scientifically analysed as bad.) He's worried that any advice that says sugar should be cut from the diet is not yet based on solid science.

Government policy based on poor science could make things worse. He quotes the example of the fat question in the US, where he worked for several years, and says the move towards low-fat products had unintended consequences. It turned out that low-fat items or the labels that say 'healthy' have done more harm than good. For a long time I bought only low-fat plain yogurt to eat for breakfast with my granola and fruit. No longer – I now only have full-fat because I learned that being swayed by low-calorie alternatives won't necessarily result in weight loss. Research has consistently shown that we tend to eat around 23 per cent more of such products because they are not as filling as those which contain fat.

An audit carried out in 2014 also found that these supposedly 'healthy' products can contain up to four times more sugar than the regular alternative, and too much sugar is definitely considered bad. Despite the lack of scientific evidence to show sugar is causing obesity, it is accepted that excessive amounts, often consumed because of high quantities added to processed foods and drinks, can contribute to raised blood sugar levels and resistance to insulin, which can lead to type 2 diabetes. Excessive amounts can also cause high blood pressure, put strain on the heart and, of course, are known to cause tooth decay.

Now we are so much better informed about genetics and metabolism, Professor Rubino insists there must be better scientific research on the impact of foods on the body. Governments, he says, should know the facts and stick to them. Indeed, there have been a number of attempts by governments to help us make decisions about what to buy and what to leave on the supermarket shelf. I've become quite obsessed with reading the food labels on every product I buy in order to check on the calories it contains. But I now learn from a recent review by Cambridge University, which compiled evidence from twenty-eight studies, that calorie labels reduce the amount consumed by, on average, 8 per cent, which is around 48 calories per meal. I guess it's a reduction, but hardly seems much of a saving when you consider a slice of bread typically contains around 90 calories. It's hard to know where to place one's trust.

The calorie question and its relationship to the 'in/out' idea of what you consume and what you expend in physical activity was put into surprising perspective in Professor Tim Spector's book *The Diet Myth*. He says that running the average body at rest with no exercise requires 1,300 calories a day, watching TV for an hour expends 60 calories and reading a chapter uses 80. I wonder what writing a chapter consumes calorie-wise? Obviously it's true that basic bodily functions and the demands made by the brain will consume a considerable amount of energy, but it seemed astonishing to me that what appears on the surface to be relaxing and doing very little requires so much. I shall feel less guilty in future about having a sit-down, watching a good programme or reading my book.

There is some evidence that the time of day we reserve for eating our meals can have an impact on whether or not we put on weight. In 2017, the Nobel Prize in Medicine and Physiology was awarded to three scientists: Jeffrey C. Hall, Michael Rosbash and Michael W. Young, for their work on understanding the function of the body clock, or the circadian rhythm. In 1984, they isolated a gene that controls the normal daily biological rhythm of the fruit fly. As a result, we learned that biological clocks exist in flies and all plants and organisms, including humans. We have all evolved to synchronize our biological rhythms to day and night. Our clock regulates behaviour, hormone levels, sleep patterns, body temperature and metabolism, among other things. It means that we are at our most alert and energetic during daylight hours, thus the rate at which we burn and use fuel is higher in the daytime than at night.

So, the time of day at which we eat is significant because if we eat late at night, just before the body and the metabolism slow down for sleep, we are more likely to store the calories than burn them. It's often been said that we should 'eat breakfast like a king, lunch like a prince and dinner like a pauper', and of course, for centuries, before electric light, life was ordered by the rising and setting of the sun, so food was cooked and eaten in daylight except in the wealthiest households where the cost of candles was not a problem.

It was a dining habit that lasted well into the twentieth century. During my childhood a big breakfast to start the day was always cooked. What we now call lunch was always referred to as dinner – just as lunchtime meals at school are still often referred to as school dinners. That was the main meal of the day. Tea was a light serving of salad or sandwiches and maybe a buttered scone, and supper was maybe a cup of Ovaltine and a biscuit. Having your large dinner in the evening is very much a modern invention. We now have reliable light in the evening, even as the days darken earlier, so we tend to work later. And that means eating later still.

It does appear to make a difference. In one study, 420 participants on a twenty-week weight-loss programme were divided into groups according to what time of day they ate their main meal. They were given exactly the same amount and type of food, and those who dined late in the day lost less weight at a slower rate than those who dined at lunchtime. It's worth considering going back to the old ways, and trying to make more of lunch and less of dinner.

Diet for Type 2 Diabetes

It's long been known that obesity leads to an increased risk of type 2 diabetes; and as levels of obesity have risen, so too has the occurrence of the disease. In 2018, around 3.5 million people were affected, at a cost to the NHS of more than £10 billion a year (in direct and indirect costs). It's a leading cause of sight loss, lower-limb amputation, kidney failure, heart attack and stroke. It's a metabolic condition caused by glucose or blood sugar levels that are too high. When you are healthy, the pancreas releases insulin to help your body store and use sugar from the food you eat. Diabetes occurs when the insulin the pancreas secretes is insufficient or the body can't recognize the insulin and use it properly. It's known as insulin resistance.

Back in the early twentieth century, before the discovery of insulin in 1922, type 1 diabetes was often a fatal disease, and type 2 was very unusual. It was known that blood sugar was a cause of the problem and it was suspected that a substance from the pancreas might be responsible for controlling it. But, before insulin was introduced, a US doctor called Frederick Allen came to the conclusion that it was a complex metabolic disease and, by experimenting with dogs and other animals, found a severe, calorie-restricted diet could help control the condition. He published his findings in 1913 and there's no doubt his methods, which did not provide a cure, saved thousands of lives long enough for the patients to benefit from the introduction of insulin.

Professor Roy Taylor of Newcastle University became fascinated by the Allen diet and wondered if it might have an application in the twenty-first century. He concentrated his research on the liver and the pancreas, and identified what he calls the twin cycle hypothesis. He found that when there was too much fat in the liver, glucose was 'slung out', as he put it to me, and the insulin couldn't cope. The other half of the twin cycle was fat in the pancreas, reducing its capacity to produce insulin.

He was aware that in the early days of bariatric surgery it had been observed that patients who had been operated on because of morbid obesity had found their type 2 diabetes went into remission. He wondered whether something along the lines of the Allen diet might produce the same results. First, in 2011, he tested fasting blood sugar levels in a small number of patients who had consumed no sugar at all for seven days – and found them to be normal. The level of fat in the pancreas and in the liver had fallen and the insulin-secretion cells in the pancreas had woken up.

He was convinced the idea was not a flash in the pan and wondered if it might be useful for the NHS if he could prove that type 2 diabetes could be put into remission in such a way. He didn't find it difficult to recruit enough patients to take part in the first trial. He selected eleven individuals who all had type 2 diabetes and weighed around 16 to 17 stone – not grossly obese, as he described them to me – used an MRI scan to meas-ure the fat in their bodies and put them on a very restricted diet.

Each day they were given three meal-replacement drinks of 200 calories each and were encouraged to eat three portions of non-starchy salads and vegetables as well. Some of the reports on the diet say 800 calories was the permitted daily allowance. Professor Taylor told me it was 700 calories. Only water – plenty of it – was to be drunk, with no poultry, fish or meat, bread or pasta, dairy (including skimmed milk), root vegetables such as potato, sweet potato or turnip, pulses, fruits and no alcohol. The diet was to continue for eight weeks.

Professor Taylor told me he was hugely surprised at the results. He'd been a doctor for forty years and was astonished to find an average weight loss of 2½ stone per patient. They said hunger had not been a problem after twenty-four hours on the regime, their blood glucose levels had returned to normal, and fat in the liver and the pancreas had reduced considerably. The cost to the NHS in the research setting with constant support, testing and advice was just over £1,000 per person – considerably less than a lifetime of treatment with prescription drugs.

The trial was extended and is now known as DiRECT – Diabetes Reduction Clinical Trial – and Professor Taylor was convinced that he could say type 2 diabetes is curable. He was careful not to overstate his success as it is, as we've seen, extremely difficult for his patients to sustain their weight loss. After one year he found fewer than half of his patients (46 per cent) were free of diabetes, and after two years just over one-third (36 per cent) were still free of the disease.

After the eight weeks on the restrictive diet, patients are helped with a stepped return to eating normally. They're advised that no fast foods must be eaten, portions must be small, and dieticians help them devise recipes and understand what foods will best help them keep their weight down and the diabetes at bay and maintain a healthy weight. For the majority, their weight began to creep up gradually, and those in difficulties were offered a rescue package of going back on the strict regime.

Professor Taylor hoped he might have had a blank slate on which to reform the way people eat, but he accepts that he hasn't solved all the problems, because food plays such an important role in our pleasure and sociability. Each patient is an individual with their own constitution, and only the most motivated and determined will succeed in keeping their weight down. Two years down the line he is not so quick to say his method provides a cure for type 2 diabetes, only that he's proved it is 'potentially reversible'.

There is another regime that reports some success in reversing the disease: the 5:2 diet devised by the BBC health journalist Dr Michael Mosley and which recommends fasting for two non-consecutive days each week. On those days women should consume only 500 calories and men 600 calories, and for the rest of the week they can eat normally. Professor Susan Jebb, a nutritional scientist at Oxford University, adapted Dr Mosley's *The Fast Diet* slightly for a television programme called *What's the Right Diet for You?* She made the two fast days consecutive and asked the dieters to consume 800 calories on those days, with minimal carbohydrates. Her theory was that on the first of the two days, much of the stored carbohydrate would be depleted, and on the second day the individual would burn fat – in effect, entering a short period of ketosis.

I haven't tried either variation of the 5:2 diet, but a very close friend, who had just been diagnosed with impaired glucose tolerance and was considered pre-diabetic, did it religiously, and her glucose tolerance became normal again. She found it an acceptable and sustainable diet as it wasn't faddy and enabled her to schedule her fasting days to suit her social life. She was still able to enjoy eating out with friends on other days of the week. She also, as a bonus, lost a stone in weight and is trying hard to keep it up.

Stigma

Rebecca Puhl is Deputy Director for the Rudd Center for Food Policy and Obesity, and a professor in the Department of Human Development and Family Studies at the University of Connecticut in the US. She is also Director of Research at the Weight Stigma Initiative at Yale. As a psychologist she has spent eighteen years studying the effects of stigma on the overweight and obese. She has found consistent evidence that it's a pervasive problem, which hurts and upsets the individual, but is rarely discussed as a legitimate problem affecting life, wellbeing and health.

She told me that the stigma has to be confronted at an early age and says children as young as three are having to deal with negative stereotypes. Even at nursery or infant school, they will find it hard to make friends. She has had such youngsters tell her that 'nobody wants to be friends with a fat person'.

More children in the US suffer from obesity than from any other chronic condition, and the UK is not far behind. One-third of US children and youths are overweight or obese, and 17 per cent of children from two to nineteen years of age are obese. Puhl quotes one study that revealed children with severe obesity had quality-of-life scores worse than children of similar ages who had cancer.

Research into the psychology of weight gain shows that children face stigma from parents and other family members, teachers, healthcare professionals and society at large, so are vulnerable to its negative consequences in school, at home and in clinical settings. It's interesting that Professor Puhl quotes a history of the way disease stigma has been perceived in the past as a legitimate barrier to prevention, intervention and treatment. Conditions such as HIV/AIDS, various cancers, alcoholism and drug use were initially stigmatized and required considerable efforts by the medical community to reduce stigma-induced barriers that impaired effective treatment.

One of Puhl's studies includes the extent to which children are vulnerable to weight stigma through the media. Her analysis of the content of popular children's books, shows and movies found they reinforce weight stigma through stereotypical portrayals of characters who appear to have larger body sizes.

Characters who are visually slim are often depicted as being kind, popular and attractive, but characters with larger body sizes are frequently aggressive, unpopular, evil, unhealthy and the target of humour or ridicule.

Given that young people spend a considerable number of hours each day reading or watching television and consuming other media, it's inevitable they are exposed to such images, and their peers, who may not be obese, see overweight characters being treated badly. It's a dangerous example for them all to follow.

It's a problem with which I suspect lots of us are familiar. In my day, it was the name of the character from a popular series of children's stories, Billy Bunter, that was thrown at any kid in the class who was a bit overweight; or maybe Tweedledum or Tweedledee, popularized by Lewis Carroll, were used to insult a podgy kid. I recall my mother using all three names on those occasions when, like so many children, I got a bit round prior to a growth spurt.

Billy Bunter was created in 1908 and remained popular until the mid-1960s. Stories featuring him were written by Charles Hamilton under the pseudonym Frank Richards, and Billy was a pupil at Greyfriars School. He was in the Lower Fourth – the Remove – implying that being dramatically overweight meant he was not very bright.

The illustrations show an extraordinarily rotund body, fat face with endless chins, specs, and tight, checked trousers enclosing his enormous legs. He was clearly intended to be a comic character, but was openly described as greedy, obtuse, lazy, deceitful, slothful, self-important and conceited. His only saving grace seemed to be that he loved his mother almost as much as his tuck.

Tweedledum and Tweedledee were tubby twins who are thought to have made their first appearance in print in the seventeenth century in an epigram referring to the disagreements between Handel and Giovanni Bononcini and written by John Byrom. The characters are best known from the perspective of nonsense comedy in *Through the Looking Glass, and What Alice Found There*.

Then, of course, there's the great Nobel Prize-winning author William Golding's classic, *Lord of the Flies*, published in 1954 and studied in English literature classes everywhere. The story, filmed in 1963 and again in 1990, involves a group of British schoolboys being shot down over a desert island during an unnamed war, choosing leaders and working together for survival. Inevitably, things deteriorate into vicious violence, and the death of several characters occurs before the boys are rescued.

One of the central characters is Piggy. He's the one who finds a conch shell and comes up with the idea of using it to make a sound, which will carry and will call the boys together. He's the intellectual among the boys, but he's plump, bespectacled, awkward and averse to physical labour because he suffers from asthma. He's dedicated to the idea of civilization, but he's killed by one of the other characters, Roger, symbolizing the triumph of brute savagery over civilized order. It's a wonderful and important novel, but did the tragic brainiac have to be called Piggy, a nickname he hated?

The stereotype in children's literature has continued unabated and we still see being fat as code for being greedy, lazy and morally corrupt. In the Harry Potter books, Dudley Dursley, Crabbe and Goyle are overweight and bullies. In Judy Blume's classic *Blubber*, published in 1974, the narrator of the story, Jill, joins her classmates in ostracizing and bullying Linda, an awkward and chubby girl who gives a 'show and tell' report to her class about whales, is subsequently nicknamed Blubber by the rest of the class and bullied physically and psychologically.

Perhaps Augustus Gloop in Roald Dahl's *Charlie and the Chocolate Factory*, in both book and film mode, is most openly ridiculed. The Oompa-Loompas sing, 'Augustus Gloop, Augustus Gloop! The great big, greedy nincompoop! Augustus Gloop, so big and vile! So greedy, foul and infantile!' Roald Dahl rather made a habit of emphasizing the size of his more unpleasant characters. Miss Trunchbull in *Matilda* is 'a formidable female, a gigantic holy terror', and the horrible Aunt Sponge in *James and the Giant Peach* is 'enormously fat and very short'.

Ursula in the popular 1989 Disney film *The Little Mermaid* is undoubtedly one of the most disturbing fat characters in children's movies. She's the one who promises to help Ariel – slim and beautiful, as most admirable characters are – achieve her ambition to become human, and sings a terrifying song in which she claims to help 'poor unfortunate souls' who are miserable, lonely and depressed. In other words, they want to become fatter if they're too thin, or thinner if they're too fat, but only if they can afford to pay the price. She fails in her attempt to ruin Ariel's life, as is the way in all fairy stories, but only at the last minute.

There have, of course, been some efforts to address the question of fat shaming in the film and television industries, with Melissa McCarthy leading the way in TV series such as *The Gilmore Girls* and films including *Bridesmaids*, *The Heat*, *Spy*, *Ghostbusters* and, most recently, *Can You Ever Forgive Me?* It is, though, still unusual to see a film with a plus-size woman in a leading role without any fat jokes and, successful though McCarthy may be, there have often been critics who have been extremely dismissive of her talent because 'she's obese'. Her recent weight loss, on the other hand, has been greatly praised.

On television, Dawn French as the vicar of Dibley was a huge step forward. Her character, Geraldine Granger, was presented as clever, funny and beautiful. The fact that she's a big woman is never ignored, but it's not presented as a barrier to her work or her love life. Geraldine is always in on any of the jokes. Then there's *My Mad Fat Diary*, based on the diary by Rae Earl. Rae is a woman who is constantly learning how to love herself and believes she can be loved in return. Her love interest loves her because he doesn't mind her weight at all and has not taken up with her as a dare or a joke, but because he truly cares for her.

The best example of a recent film that appeals to young people is *Booksmart*, which came out in 2019. Kaitlyn Dever (slim) plays Amy, and Beanie Feldstein (not slim) plays Molly. They are best friends who've neglected their social lives in favour of academic study. On the night of their high-school graduation they realize they maybe should have worked less and played more. They set out on a wild night of partying and no reference is ever made to either girl being more or less attractive because of her size. They remain best friends.

Professor Puhl recommends complaining to editors, writers or producers where unhelpful characterizations are promoted. She also urges that care should be taken in the use of language. She wants to encourage teachers and health professionals to use appropriate and sensitive vocabulary when discussing weight with young people, families and other members of a healthcare team, as words can heal or harm.

Recent research shows that terms such as 'weight' and 'body mass index' are preferred by adolescents who are overweight and obese, whereas 'obese', 'extremely obese', 'fat' or 'weight problem' induce feelings of sadness, embarrassment and shame, particularly if such words are used by a parent. She also recommends the use of what's known as 'people first' language. In other words it places the individual first, rather than the disease or disability, thus 'a child with obesity' rather than 'an obese child'.

Adolescents can have a particularly hard time. In 2011, Puhl asked 1,555 students from two high schools in Central Connecticut to report any experience of weight-based teasing and bullying at school. Only those who said they had already been victimized because of their weight were to be included in the study. Of the 1,555 asked about victimization, 394 came forward and said they had been abused because of their weight. Fifty-six per cent were female, 84 per cent were Caucasian, and their average age was 16.4 years. She discovered that half of the sample felt sad and depressed. They felt bad about their bodies, but worse about themselves and how they had come to be so fat. They were angry, and some said they often felt afraid.

Both boys and girls were likely to use coping strategies of avoidance, particularly failing to attend any gym classes, and they also comforted themselves with increased food consumption and binge eating. The number of students who were skipping school or reporting that their grades were harmed because of weight-based teasing went up by 5 per cent per incident, even after controlling for gender, race, age, grades and weight status.

Adolescents from the original group of 1,555 were asked to report what they observed about how weight was used to discriminate against their overweight peers and 84 per cent said they had seen them being teased in a mean way, particularly during physical activities, and a slightly smaller percentage said their overweight and obese peers had been ignored, avoided, excluded from social activities, had negative rumours spread about them and were teased in the cafeteria. Most of the students reported they had witnessed verbal threats and physical harassment towards the obese, and some said they felt comfortable stepping in to help an overweight peer who had been teased, but a good number simply remained passive bystanders.

As far as obese adults are concerned, Puhl's research has found that weight-based stigma, prejudice and outright discrimination are rampant. One review of studies showed that 19 per cent of adults with class I obesity (a BMI of 30–35) reported experiencing treatment they viewed as unfair in various settings, and the figure rose to 42 per cent for people who were more obese. At each level of obesity, women reported more discrimination than men.

The rise in obesity rates, which means almost 40 per cent of Americans are now classed as obese, and 28.7 per cent of people in England, has not reduced the stigma. Overtly negative attitudes towards people based on body weight had declined by only 15 per cent from 2004 to 2016. In contrast, explicit racism dropped by 37 per cent and explicit anti-gay feelings by nearly half. When researchers examined 'implicit' bias – unconsciously held attitudes, which are revealed through laboratory testing – weight bias, unlike every other type, appeared to be getting slightly worse over time.

Professor Puhl says it's not surprising that such bias often translates into the mistreatment of people. One review of existing research found statistically significant penalties for people who are overweight or obese at every step of the employment process: hiring, evaluations, promotion and firing, and most studies are consistent that there's also a wage penalty.

The Borgata Hotel Casino and Spa in Atlantic City obsessively monitored the weight of its waitresses, according to twenty-two of them who attempted to sue their employer in 2008. They had been told they would be suspended if their weight went up by 7 per cent from when they were first hired. A New Jersey judge threw out the case, explaining that state law was silent about weight discrimination. There was an appeal, but the state supreme court agreed with the decision of the first judge three years previously.

Professor Puhl gave me a number of examples of weight discrimination being used by employers quite openly. One woman, a public-relations professional, explained how her supervisor made her undergo humiliating weekly weigh-ins in his office to keep her job. A hospital in Victoria, Texas, made headlines in 2012 after it imposed a strict body-mass limit on employees. A BMI of 35 was the cut-off point and administrators said the decision was based on patients' expectations of what a healthcare provider should look like. The rule was clearly discriminatory, but entirely legal.

Massachusetts has a bill that specifically makes weight discrimination illegal. It's very concise, adding weight and height to the list of protected categories in existing anti-discrimination law, alongside race, age, sexuality and disability. Michigan's Civil Rights Law has prohibited weight discrimination for more than forty years, but it's rare, even in the litigation culture of the US, to find such redress open to people who have suffered discrimination because of their weight.

The law in the UK was tested in 2015 in *Bickerstaff* v. *Butcher* in the Northern Ireland Industrial Tribunal. The Equality Act of 2010 does not specifically include obesity as a protected condition, but in the Bickerstaff case, a ruling from the European Court of Justice was referred to in support of Mr Bickerstaff, who said he was harassed by his colleagues because of his weight. The ECJ ruling in the case of a Danish child-minder, Karsten Kaltoft, who claimed he was sacked for being too fat, concluded that 'if obesity hinders full and effective participation at work it could count as a disability'. Disability is protected under the Equality Act and Mr Bickerstaff won his case.

As Professor Puhl says, it's often assumed that calling attention to people's weight in a negative context will motivate them to adopt an exercise regime or otherwise improve their health. In fact, the research suggests the opposite, and the obese who suffer such stigma are frequently too afraid even to see their doctor for help and advice, for fear of being told off. Weight stigma worsens people's quality of life, even increasing mortality rates, often because of factors such as increased stress and depression.

Sceptics who resist the introduction of anti-weight-discrimination laws use the argument that, unlike race, age or gender, weight is largely under the control of the individual, ignoring the genetic and environmental factors which, as we have seen, are prominent contributors to obesity. They say anti-weight-discrimination laws could make it illegal for a company to encourage weight loss among employees in an effort to reduce insurance costs. Puhl argues that it's easy to introduce a non-discriminatory wellness programme to promote healthy behaviour for all workers, rather than penalizing one group.

Professor Puhl concluded our discussion about stigma thus: 'Weight discrimination is a legitimate and prevalent societal problem. It inflicts pain and suffering, causes financial harm and impairs quality of life. It should be banned, just like other forms of invidious discrimination.'

Fear of Food

It seems to me that the most important lesson we learn from understanding the science that's known thus far about food and obesity is that we need to really make the effort to truly comprehend this: the research makes it absolutely clear that we put on weight for all kinds of reasons not associated with laziness, greed or lack of moral fibre. We need to spread this message far and wide.

Nor should we demonize, fear or exclude any food groups from our diet unless a doctor specifically advises it because of a particular condition. We should eat in moderation, choosing smaller portions than we may have had in the past, but never feeling guilty about a few chips from time to time, or the occasional, delicious chocolate eclair. It's just food and it's pleasurable. The old advert for fresh cream cakes, 'naughty but nice', is so yesterday. Nice, yes; naughty, no.

Portions are what really matter. Studies suggest that if a reduction in exposure to larger-size food portions, packages and tableware could be achieved, the daily consumption of energy, based on the typical UK diet, could be reduced by between 144 and 228 calories per person. Too much of anything, whether it's meat, fat, sugar, fruit or even vegetables, is bad, and too little of anything, even sugar and fat, is also bad. Remember the science and eat accordingly when you're hungry. And, as Susie Orbach whispered, metaphorically, so often in my ear, 'Listen to your appetite, and when it tells you you're full, stop.'

Of course, psychologically speaking, it's not all that easy. For years and years I continued to try to make a joke of her whisperings. It wasn't really funny, but I always said, as I'm sure you may have, and as I explained earlier, 'Ah, yes, Susie, that's all very well, but it's the one subject on which I appear to be profoundly deaf.'

9

The Fat Chance

It was, finally, sheer desperation that drove me to take the final fat chance, which I accept will not be the weight-loss solution for everyone. But for me, after years of thinking about it and fearing it, metabolic surgery became my only way out of the state in which I found myself.

There I was, in late 2014, sixty-four years old, ranging in weight from 22 to 24 stone and with a BMI between 45 and 50 – well into the obese range, if not, indeed, morbidly obese. I was depressed and almost at the end of my tether, having tried so many diets and failed, failed and failed again to lose weight. Well, no, actually, I'd frequently succeeded in losing the weight, but had found it impossible to sustain once I considered the diet to be over because I'd reached my goal. Then, time and again, as I relaxed into not being on a diet and began to think I could enjoy food again, I consistently discovered I weighed even more than I had before.

I didn't understand the science then, but I knew the risks to which I was exposing myself before my son Charlie delivered his devastatingly accurate assessment of the future that lay in store for me: the massively obese woman on the mobility scooter, slowly doing her circuit of the park with her little dogs trotting alongside, leads attached to the handlebars.

'That, Mum, before very long, is going to be you.' I knew he was right and that I could look forward to an even more severe disability or worse.

I knew type 2 diabetes can develop frequently as a result of obesity and that it can lead to blindness and, in the most extreme cases, loss of circulation and then to the amputation of toes or even a leg. I was also risking heart failure or a stroke. My beloved, obese maternal grandmother had a stroke in her mid-seventies and died within twenty-four hours. In some ways she was lucky to go as quickly as she did. She would have hated to suffer the typical results of such a condition – loss of movement, loss of speech, and becoming completely dependent on carers to cater for her every need. For far too long I allowed myself to be scared that I would share her fate, without doing anything about it.

I had a number of friends and colleagues who had gone down the gastric band route. The TV and radio presenters Vanessa Feltz, Jay Hunt and Fern Britton had all lost significant amounts of weight by having the band surgically placed around their stomach to make it impossible to eat to excess, but I was cautious, as was my husband and the rest of my family. We'd all heard horror stories about bad experiences of cheap gastric band deals performed abroad, others where the gastric band had stretched and food consumption and weight had gone up, and others still where the patient was so desperate to consume the 'treats' they loved that they melted chocolate and other sweet things in order to get them past the band.

Equally, the result of the gastric band experience where weight loss had been successful had not been reported to me as pleasant. The band merely made it impossible to consume innumerable foods as it served only to restrict the amount of food a banded stomach could hold. I remember bumping into Vanessa in the street and her telling me how she could no longer eat one of her favourite foods, a bagel with smoked salmon and cream cheese, even in the tiniest quantities. She longed for it, dreamed about it, her appetite was undiminished and she felt almost permanently hungry. The band had no impact on the hunger hormones, which seemed to rage pretty constantly. It was just like being permanently on the faddiest of diets. It was not a foolproof method for weight loss.

Another reason I was held back from signing up to any form of surgical intervention was the fact that I'd had so many operations as a result of the breast cancer and the wrecked hips. I think the family was frightened that my luck might run out this time and I would be sure to die under an anaesthetic. It was during my recovery from the hip replacement that I'd heard of the tragic death of the film director Anthony Minghella, who never woke up from an operation to remove a cancerous growth on his neck. His experience made me sad and scared of surgery too.

It seems obvious to me now that my family also seriously believed that I could still achieve weight loss, not by faddy or crash dieting, but in the traditional way by accepting that it was simply a case of less energy in and more out, and applying will-power (of which I seemed to have plenty when it came to going to work and running a family). They were so wrong, but it was some time before I learned how wrong they were and why.

Like them, though, I was extremely worried about the state of my health, and was becoming increasingly disabled. I began to dread my walks in the park or in the countryside with my dogs, knowing every step would be agonizingly painful as my back and knees were giving me serious gyp, and that we would have to stop frequently at every bench that came our way. Nevertheless, I avoided going to the GP to discuss my weight, so I learned from personal experience that the stigma of obesity can hold back even the most seemingly intelligent and confident person from seeking medical help in case they face censure rather than sensibility.

I couldn't avoid seeing the new GP for a check-up to discuss my asthma treatment and my post-breast-cancer medication, though, which was ongoing nearly ten years after the mastectomy. That was when he said, 'I think it's time you did something about your weight.' I explained my disastrous history of dieting and he, rather sympathetically I have to say, suggested what he described as a 'new kind of surgical treatment – a gastric balloon'.

The procedure is not strictly surgical and doesn't involve a general anaesthetic. There is sedation to enable the insertion of the balloon through the mouth, the gullet and into the stomach. Once in the stomach it's inflated and filled with sterile saline. The procedure takes around ten minutes and it's only necessary to spend an hour or two in the hospital. Possible side effects include nausea, bloating and stomach cramps, and the follow-up care period is designed to help patients develop a healthy relationship with food, where they eat the right things at the right time for the right reasons for the rest of their lives. It includes cognitive behavioural therapy sessions to help patients change their attitude to food and end a cycle of yo-yo dieting. The balloon can be left in place for six months or a year before it's removed.

I was far from convinced it would be the answer to my considerable problems. As I read about the procedure, it seemed to be designed primarily for people who were only a stone or two overweight. I needed something much more drastic. It also made no real sense to me as, like the surgical gastric band, it would have no impact on the hunger hormones. If it were to be removed after six months, as my GP had suggested, would I not find myself in exactly the same position as when I'd succeeded in achieving a great deal of weight loss after following a strict diet, where I'd just be raging with hunger again and would simply put the weight, and more, back on? I was not prepared to give it a go and risk feeling a failure again.

The first step towards my decision to make further investigations into what's generally known as bariatric surgery – from the Greek *baros*, meaning weight – came as a result of an interview I conducted with Dr Billy White, a young surgeon at University College Hospital in London. We were discussing obesity in children and his work as a surgeon carrying out bariatric operations on young people, often in their early teens. He had even treated children as young as nine who had already developed type 2 diabetes as a result of their obesity – a problem we now know is rising in numbers among youngsters all the time. When we'd finished the interview and were chatting after the programme, I asked him, with one of those silly, slightly embarrassed grins on my face, what help he would recommend for a middle-aged, verging on old, obese woman.

'If you really want to know,' he said, 'let's not discuss it here at your place of work. Here's my email, think about it and, if you want to pursue it further, we'll meet for a coffee and I'll talk you through it.'

I emailed him the very next day. We met that afternoon for coffee, and for the first time I began to hear about the progress in scientific knowledge about what causes obesity, why it can be so easy to put on weight and so difficult to lose it, and what is involved in the different surgical procedures designed to help with what he called 'the disease of obesity'. That was the first time I had heard it described as a disease. I listened carefully to everything he had to say.

He explained there were two types of bariatric surgery, which he considered might be suitable for me. Both are performed under general anaesthetic, using laparoscopic (i.e. keyhole) methods. It means the surgeon doesn't have to open you up completely and leave you with a large and unsightly scar. He or she makes small incisions in the abdomen and inserts a flexible viewing tube to see inside while the operation is performed.

The first and more radical option is called a gastric bypass. Surgical staples are used to create a small pouch at the top of the stomach, and the pouch is then connected to the small intestine, bypassing the rest of the stomach. It therefore takes less food to make you feel full and fewer calories are absorbed from the food you eat.

The alternative is a sleeve gastrectomy; where a large part of the stomach – 75–80 per cent – is completely removed so that it's much smaller than before. As with the bypass, you can't eat as much as you used to and you feel full sooner. The old stomach could contain around 1.5 litres but after surgery, only around 300 millilitres. The advantage with the sleeve, it seemed to me, was that there is no interference in the normal journey of food and drink through the digestive system. The now smaller, sleeve-like stomach is stitched together with surgical staples, but essentially remains intact, with the oesophagus at the top and the small intestine at the bottom, just as it had been before the operation. Billy told me there was less risk of any complications with the sleeve gastrectomy than with the bypass, and even drew me pictures on the back of a serviette.

Most importantly, he gave me the name of the doctor he recommended to carry out the procedure. Professor Francesco Rubino, based at King's College Hospital in South London. He was the first doctor in this country to be appointed professor of what he calls metabolic (not bariatric) surgery. According to Billy, he was the best. Not only was he a brilliant surgeon, but he was at the forefront of scientific research into obesity and metabolic disorders such as type 2 diabetes. Billy gave me his phone number.

I dillied and dallied about calling, wondering if I really could face what Billy had made sound so easy and straightforward, but I knew would mean lots of tests, visits to the hospital, a long wait for surgery on the NHS, a short period as an in-patient, and then goodness knows what it would be like once the die had been cast and I had had half my stomach removed irreversibly.

A week or so later I had dinner with a friend who was a producer on one of Radio 4's investigative documentary strands. I told her about Billy White's advice and she lit up with excitement. 'Oh,' she said, 'I know Professor Rubino. We made a programme about how slow the NHS has been to finance metabolic surgery for obesity. We interviewed him. There's clear evidence that the operations can reverse type 2 diabetes, help the grossly obese lose weight and improve their health in so many ways. And it saves the NHS a fortune.

'We worked out that this type of surgery pays for itself within three years by saving on prescriptions for the treatment of diabetes and blood glucose monitoring, and improved physical activity helps patients return to work and reduces the need for disability benefits. It's a no-brainer. It's a treatment for an increasingly common disease, which saves lives and money. Go for it!'

I made the call. Professor Rubino could not have been kinder or more welcoming. He invited me to meet him one evening in the part of the hospital where he carries out his research, and I knew from the moment I sat across the desk from him that I had met the man who would change my life. For the first time ever I was talking to a true expert who was telling me that, yes, I may be obese, but it was not my fault.

In his charming Italian accent he began to explain the complexity of body weight, how it's tied in to hormones and genetics, and is not nearly so simple as energy in and energy out. It's not true for everyone, he said, that eating less and exercising more will lead to weight loss. Some of his patients, suffering from clinical obesity, could be made to walk around the world being force-fed a healthy diet and it wouldn't begin to touch their problem. 'Forty per cent of the population,' he told me, 'has a serious disease. And, yes, I do frame it as a disease. So many patients have a poor quality of life. They have sleep apnoea, diabetes, mobility problems and, I assure you, anyone with a BMI over 40 will not be able to cure the disease by themselves.'

I can't begin to tell you how my spirits were lifted by this warm, gentle, knowledgeable scientist telling me I was not greedy or lazy, but I had a problem with my metabolism. What a relief it was to have it confirmed that my growing understanding of how the metabolism reacts to the dieting rollercoaster was correct. Dieting causes obesity, he continued. As do the fashions for super-size meals, sugary drinks, wine o'clock and our devotion to the motor car and neglect of Shanks' pony, the simple act of walking. He was critical of the food industry, which he blames for causing the obesity epidemic, but he was not altogether damning. It was at this first encounter that he told me the food industry did not deliberately set out to make us fatter, but that in the process of trying to help eradicate inadequate nutrition they had introduced preservatives to ensure food remained safe to eat for longer, and salt and sugar to make it taste good.

He worries that policymakers are involved in making decisions that are not always based on fact. He wants more scientific research to inform us which foods are dangerous and which are not. Bad science, he says, leads to unintended consequences, and health ministries should only stick to proven scientific facts in giving their advice on nutrition.

We talked about how he came to this kind of work. He did his basic medical training in Italy, became a general surgical registrar in Rome and had no interest in bariatric surgery. Indeed, he resisted any efforts among his superiors to persuade him to give it a go. He, like so many others, thought people caused the problem themselves, that chopping away part of the stomach sounded barbaric and just gave obese people an easy way out, allowing them to be less responsible. For a short time he worked in France and then was offered a job in the US. It was in both countries that he studied laparoscopic surgical techniques. He became interested in the impact of surgery on type 2 diabetes when he was working as a research fellow in New York. In June 1999 he had what he describes as his eureka moment and changed his attitude completely.

He had been studying a complex bariatric procedure known as biliopancreatic diversion and went to the medical library to review the literature, hoping to explore ways in which existing surgical techniques might be improved by using staples rather than stitches. He didn't find the answers to his technical surgical questions, but he found an interesting report that said these operations were improving diabetes in 80–90 per cent of cases.

Even patients who had been on insulin found their control of blood sugars became normal without any medication after surgery. Professor Rubino realized that what he'd read presented far too striking an effect to have taken place purely by weight loss. In a substantial number of the patients – at least a third – the effect happened rapidly, in a matter of days or weeks. In such a short time there had not been much loss of weight.

He told me how excited he'd been at his discovery. 'What if the surgery itself influences diabetes directly, I wondered? I couldn't sleep that night. You don't learn in medical school that diabetes can go away, you learn that it is progressive and irreversible.' He recalled from his studies in Rome that the intestine produces hormones called incretins that spur the production of insulin. 'They're signals produced in response to food passing through the bowel,' he explained. 'They tell the pancreas the food is coming down and it's time to produce insulin to control blood sugar levels. I began to understand that surgery can alter a dysfunctional homeostatic system.'

When he reviewed the literature, he found only one paper that made the same connection and, with that exception, he said, the idea was completely heretical. Nobody wanted to know. He and his colleagues felt the theory merited a clinical trial, but it turned out the time wasn't right; people weren't ready. They submitted a proposal to the institutional review body, but it was never approved. He continued his research on diabetic rats with promising results and, when his fellowship in the US ended, he carried on his research in Strasbourg,

France. His experiments produced the first evidence that there are mechanisms independent of weight that will control diabetes when gastrointestinal surgery is performed.

He had difficulty getting his paper published. 'We sent it to major journals and the scepticism was palpable. You could feel that the idea was still too far away. But once the paper eventually came out, it inspired other surgeons, particularly in South America and India. They took the idea and ran with it. They did the same operation on humans and from there they reported early data showing that these patients could enjoy improvement of diabetes and at times complete resolution.'

In March 2007, Professor Rubino organized the first International Consensus Conference on Gastrointestinal Surgery for the Treatment of Type 2 Diabetes in Rome. He describes it as an historic moment. 'Immediately after that,' he says, 'five or six professional societies changed their name from bariatric to metabolic.'

I did not have type 2 diabetes, but I had been diagnosed with glucose resistance and would, had I continued to be so obese, inevitably have developed it. The idea of the surgery became an increasingly attractive option as Professor Rubino and I discussed in ever more detail the impact it would have on my future health. I think what impressed me most was his willingness to give as much time as was needed to make sure I understood what I would be letting myself in for.

The most significant part of our conversation was the information about why surgery, either a sleeve or a bypass, was so much more effective for weight loss and keeping diabetes at bay than any other plan, such as Professor Roy Taylor's 700-calorie-a-day diet. As Professor Rubino pointed out, the diet method was actually quite an expensive commitment for the NHS, as diet shakes had to be provided to ensure patients received the right nutrients for survival, and careful monitoring had to continue even after the eight-week diet period had ended.

He agreed that what he described as a starvation diet would help with diabetes and some patients would lose weight, but he found it unlikely that it would be a feasible long-term solution for the morbidly obese. The low-calorie diet would create more hunger as the hormonal system began to kick into starvation mode, and patients would find it difficult to deal with feeling ravenous for much of the time. Metabolic energy would fall and patients, he believed, would struggle to stick with the plan. His main worry was that such a diet reinforces stigma as it requires patients to exercise ruthless self-control – the kind that few people have, obese or otherwise.

I learned why surgery prevents that nagging hunger hormone, ghrelin, from pestering you as you begin to lose weight. It is produced principally in the part of the stomach which is removed in the sleeve operation, which means the regulation of hunger and satiety is not left to chance. The sophisticated metabolic mechanism is changed. As the prof put it: 'It resets the software that's embedded into the system.'

He was concerned that policymakers would seize on Professor Taylor's methods, which seemed such an apparently simple method of dealing with diabetes, to the detriment of those doctors who were trying to persuade them that metabolic surgery should be endorsed as a tried-and-tested method of dealing with the diabetes and obesity crises. He continues to be frustrated at those doctors, politicians and media who fail to understand the benefits of the surgery, its potential in the long term to save the health service money, and who continue to assume it's just an easy way out for the greedy and lazy.

He suspects there's a reluctance, particularly on the part of politicians, to be seen to be spending money on people they consider to be fat, gluttonous and idle. Ideas about obesity prevail, despite being formed in the Middle Ages, when gluttony and idleness were classed among the seven deadly sins, and he believes it's time twenty-first-century scientific understanding should inform decision-makers rather than ancient myth.

Professor Rubino continues to hold conferences on progress in research and knowledge about the effectiveness of the surgical option, to which he invites the media and policymakers. He finds it hard to understand why no one questions investment in the surgical treatment of cancer or any other serious condition, but obesity, also a dangerous, expensive and potentially killer disease, continues to be underfunded.

My weight and BMI of 45 qualified me for treatment on the NHS. The National Institute for Health and Care Excellence (NICE) recommends that surgery should be provided if you have a BMI of 40 or more, or one between 35 and 40 together with a serious condition that might improve if you were to lose weight, such as type 2 diabetes or high blood pressure. You have to be able to show you've tried other weight-loss methods, such as dieting and exercise, but have struggled to lose weight or keep it off. You have to agree to long-term follow-up after surgery, seeing a nutritionist, making healthy lifestyle changes and attending regular check-ups. Treatment on the NHS is a bit of a postcode lottery, with different areas imposing different criteria, so it's recommended that you check with your GP if you think surgery might be an answer for you.

Professor Rubino and I agreed that a sleeve gastrectomy would be the best option for me. We ruled out gastric bands because of the known problems there have been with discomfort and stretching of the band. We also ruled out a gastric bypass. The sleeve would not disrupt the natural flow of the small amount of food the new stomach could accommodate. Unlike the band or the balloon it would be irreversible, permanently reducing the volume of my stomach.

He signed me up as a patient on his NHS list. I next saw him in his clinic where we did blood tests – no type 2, blood pressure surprisingly normal – and the BMI calculation. The imperial formula is weight (lb)/[height (in)]^2 × 703 – yes, it's complicated. My maths wouldn't allow me even to comprehend the equation, let alone work it out, but there are handy calculators on the internet. It's a formula developed by a US insurance company in the 1940s to determine what they considered to be an ideal weight. If your BMI was over what they considered acceptable, your premiums went up. It is, says the professor, an unreliable measurement for surgery. He quotes the members of the England rugby team as examples, who would have tremendously high BMIs but are all muscle and as fit as fleas. Some super-heavy people, he says, are super-healthy. It's the different body mechanisms that count and he believes that someone with a BMI of 30 who has type 2 diabetes should have surgery, but won't get it. The NHS insists on its strict criteria.

Once we had agreed on my treatment progressing on the NHS, I started on the one-year course known as the Tier 3 weight-management programme as described by Jools and her support group in Chapter 7. It has to be completed before you can be put on the Tier 4 bariatric surgery service and the waiting list. It's a long pathway that involves meetings with psychologists, nutritionists and a weight-loss support group. If you gain any weight or fail to attend any of your appointments, you're effectively thrown off the programme and returned to your GP.

Professor Rubino considers it a waste of money and time, as delaying surgery in patients who have diabetes risks the operation being less effective. The reasoning behind the tiers is the NHS's idea that 'we need to spend more on prevention', but as the prof explained, prevention applies to healthy people. Anyone approved even to begin the treatment process is, by definition, unhealthy. Weight loss and change in lifestyle, he believes, will not be achieved by the long wait and it doesn't save the NHS from having to spend on those who are sick.

By that point I had learned enough about why I was so fat and what was necessary to fix it, so I made the decision to walk away from the NHS and proceed privately. I had just turned sixty-five; I knew no diet or exercise programme, or meetings with dieticians or psychologists, was going to be effective for me in the long term; and I certainly felt that, at my age, I couldn't afford to wait another year with the threat of developing type 2 diabetes hanging over my head. My health insurance refused to pay for 'weight-loss surgery', which seems crazy to me as there's no doubt the surgery would save many more further claims in the future. Luckily, though, I had inherited a bit of money after the death of my parents. I reckoned my mother would consider it the best £11,000 she or I had ever spent.

There is an element of irony in the fact she would

undoubtedly have approved of me spending a significant portion of my inheritance on weight-loss surgery. I doubt she ever even considered her role in my struggles with my weight and the way I looked, but she would have been delighted to have a thinner daughter.

Professor Rubino fixed my surgery for Wednesday, 17 June 2015 at 5 p.m. For two weeks before the big day I was told to follow a strict 800- to 1,000-calories-a-day diet – a bit of carbohydrate, some lean fish or meat, some fruit and veg and plenty of fluids, all spread at regular intervals throughout the day. No booze and no pigging out on a last big meal the night before the operation. The aim of the diet was to reduce the size of the liver, the large organ which lies over the stomach in the abdomen. The strict regime would reduce the amount of glycogen, water and fatty deposits in the liver and make it easier for the surgeon to move it aside during the operation.

King's College Hospital is at the opposite end of the capital from my London home, but I have a very good friend, Ysanne, who lives close to it. She, like me, has little dogs and agreed to look after mine whilst I was in hospital, as David was working up North. She invited me to stay for two nights before admission, as I would have to go to the clinic for tests on the Tuesday. I think it's the only occasion ever I've spent time in her house when we've eaten so little and drunk absolutely nothing but water and coffee. It's very important to have sympathetic and supportive friends at such a time. I was terrified.

The Guthrie Wing of King's College Hospital is housed in what I suspect was the original part of the Victorian building before it grew with modern structures over the huge site it now occupies in Denmark Hill. As a long-standing supporter of and advocate for the NHS, I felt considerable guilt at entering such a small, quiet, exclusive little place. No queues, no bustle, just a courteous and friendly receptionist who checked me in and directed me to my room.

What luxury. Bed, chairs, table, own bathroom, but curiously I missed being in an open ward. So often, during my cancer treatment and previous surgeries for hips and a broken humerus, I've found great comfort in being able to share anxieties with fellow patients, even if some of them did tend to keep you awake all night with their snoring or complaints. Here I felt completely alone with my worries.

The nurses were attentive. The anaesthetist came at 4 p.m. and managed to make me laugh. Professor Rubino, the busiest of busy men, popped in to say hello and in no time at all I was being wheeled down to the operating theatre. Just before the anaesthetist came to knock me out, the prof came for another quick chat and asked me who I would like him to inform to let them know the op had been successful. I was astonished that he should be so willing to take the trouble to make a call in the evening and gave him Charlie's phone number, as he was the only member of the family in London at the time. 'If it were my mother undergoing surgery, I would want to know immediately that all had gone well,' he said.

From that point I remember nothing after the instruction to count. I think I got as far as two and the next thing I recall was waking up in bed in my room with Charlie standing by my bedside. I'd been in theatre for two hours and woke three hours after I'd begun to recover, so it must have been soon after 10 p.m. that I was cogent enough to register my amazement that the surgeon had made the call and Charlie had crossed London and found his way to my bed so that I would wake to the familiar face of someone I loved. I was immeasurably grateful, but I wasn't much company for him. I fell asleep again pretty quickly.

The following morning I was fully awake quite early as is always the case with hospital routines. I was not at all hungry, but I was thirsty. Only clear liquids were allowed so I had a cup of black coffee. It went down well and tasted great. It was a huge relief that I could still taste something good and keep it down. I got up feeling slightly wobbly after the anaesthetic and post-operative painkillers, but I had a shower and sat in the bedside chair feeling astonished at how little pain there was. Nothing more than the kind of rumbling you might experience with an empty stomach. And that's the way it continued, with me taking nothing more than a couple of paracetamol with some water. Of course, I had a look to see what the damage to my skin was. There were five tiny wounds, and the scars are now barely perceptible.

Lunchtime came around and I was offered a bowl of thin tomato soup. I managed about half of it. That was to be the pattern for the next two weeks. I was instructed that I should follow a liquid-only diet, consisting of protein drinks made with skimmed milk, some soups and a multivitamin. It's quite frightening because you really don't know what your new stomach can take.

I spent Thursday night in the hospital and was then declared fit to go home by Professor Rubino. Charlie came to collect me. We picked up the dogs from Ysanne's and were all astonished at the speed of my recovery and the fact that by that point I had absolutely no pain.

Once the two weeks of liquids only were over, I was instructed by the hospital's dietician to begin to introduce sloppy purées made with meat or fish and vegetables. By the time I returned to work on 1 July, only two weeks after the operation, I had moved on to purées and had a skinny latte for breakfast in the office. By 8 July I had managed to acquire two tickets for Wimbledon. I took Ysanne with me as she's the tennis tournament's number-one fan and she certainly deserved a big thank-you present for all the support she'd given me. She was beside herself with joy. I was amazed at how well I felt and how easily I was coping. I didn't even miss the strawberries and cream. I just didn't fancy them.

Eight weeks after the op I began to eat normally, ensuring I stopped the moment I began to feel full. Everything I'd learned about the hunger hormones turned out to be true. I began to feel a bit hungry at mealtimes, but was soon satisfied. The weight loss began immediately. At my first post-operative check-up, Professor Rubino warned me not to become obsessed with daily checks on the weight scales. It was hard to resist, but I did wait for a few weeks. The result was an astonishing delight. Two stone had simply fallen away. The weight loss had begun to slow by Christmas, but already 5 stone were gone and my surgeon reckoned I might lose another 4 or 5 by the summer. That would be nearly 10 stone gone in a year. Amazing!

I was soon able to go out to dinner with friends. I would order two starter-size courses and by December, celebrating a friend's birthday, I managed a salad with beetroot and blue cheese, and then a small fillet steak with green beans and a spoonful of coleslaw. I had no bread, no pudding and a small glass of red wine. I did pinch two of my friend's chips, enjoyed the meal and the company hugely, and stopped eating when I felt I'd had enough. Finally, I was listening to my appetite.

On a work day I would have a small portion of porridge with fruit and two skinny lattes at the office for breakfast. Charlie would often come round with a cheese-and-ham baguette for lunch and I would eat the two small ends. He never did like crusts. For dinner I would eat a small portion of fish or maybe some home-made shepherd's pie with a variety of vegetables and a piece of fruit. I continued taking the multi-vitamin. It was enough.

Unsurprisingly, the weight loss did wonders for my energy levels and mobility. About a month before my first Christmas following the surgery, my number-one son, Ed, suggested we take the dogs out for a walk on a chilly Saturday morning. Both my boys had long made it a mission to get me out doing some form of exercise, invariably expecting me to pull a face, finally agree and then insist on a short route, on the flat, with plenty of benches for a rest.

On this occasion we set off without any complaint from me. We went to the woods with three little dogs dancing around in delight. We came to a steep hillock. 'It's OK, Mum,' said thoughtful Ed. 'There's a way round it on the flat. You don't have to climb the hill.'

'No,' I replied, 'it's OK. There'll be a nice view from the top.'

When we reached the summit he was astonished. 'Gosh, Mum, you made it. No complaints. No breathlessness. No begging to sit down. No whingeing. This is great.'

The entire family was beginning to realize that, however daunting it had seemed at the outset, the surgery had been exactly the right thing for me.

And so we came to my first Christmas. The four of us – husband, two sons and me – stayed in our old family home in the Peak District where we lit the fires and hoped for some snow. Just enough to make the stunning landscape look pretty, but not enough to block the roads. I ordered all the basics – turkey, sprouts, pudding, brandy for the sauce, cake and mince pies (I've never been able to make them the way my mother and grandmother did). The cooking of Christmas dinner would, as always, be a shared endeavour, with the boys being such wonderful cooks.

We would sit down to the usual splendid feast, but I didn't feel the slightest bit hard done by, having to stick to smaller portions. Why would I when a smaller plateful tastes just as good as a larger one and the celebration is all about delicious, familiar flavours, eating together around an elegantly dressed table and feeling full, which for me would happen very quickly?

I had a thin slice of lean turkey breast with no crispy skin, one roast potato, a couple of sprouts, a teaspoon of stuffing, a smidgeon of cranberry sauce and just a drop of gravy. My portion of pudding was doll-size – just a tablespoon – with a drop of brandy sauce. At teatime I had a sliver of cake with a few crumbs of cheese – my Yorkshire heritage will always insist on cheese to accompany fruit cake – and I saved my mince pie for Boxing Day: just the one. I had neither the desire nor the space for chocolates.

There was no champagne. Fizzy wine or sparkling water doesn't agree with a new stomach and the other members of the family have never much liked it anyway. A glass of good red wine and tap water was fine. You might imagine such a Spartan affair would put a dampener on proceedings but, on the contrary, it's the way the new portion-conscious me wants to eat. There is no sense of deprivation, and the fact that at that point I was already 5½ stone lighter than I had been the previous year was ample cause for celebration. I was conscious that there was no more threat of type 2 diabetes, there would be no more feeling like a beached whale in an outsize swimsuit at the pool, and no more concerned comments from my husband and sons.

After lunch I didn't slump in front of the television with a box of chocolates as had been my wont. Instead, I hit the hills with the dogs because my energy levels had been transformed. As we headed towards the New Year and looked back on the previous one, I could only feel immense relief that I'd taken that scary step, and when it came to thinking about New Year resolutions, for the first time in an awfully long while I didn't have to put 'go on a diet' on the list.

Four years on and my weight appears to have stabilized at just under 14 stone. There is, I'm told, a theory called the 'set point', which says that 'in adult individuals body weight is maintained at a relatively stable level for long periods. The set-point theory suggests that body weight is regulated at a predetermined or preferred level by a feedback control mechanism.' It is, though, not fully understood how our biological systems maintain an inherited optimal-weight set point, nor how it can go so drastically wrong in cases of anorexia, bulimia or obesity. It is believed, though, that metabolic surgery helps to reset a point at which one's body is programmed to function at its best, and will fight to maintain that weight range.

So, I think that my body is now content to fluctuate between 14 and 14½ stone and I'm happy to be set at that point. I could make the effort to lose more weight, as Emma Burnell has done since her surgery by following the Slimming World regime. Emma, though, at forty-four, is much younger than me and it's generally accepted that we put on a little weight as we get older. Maybe I could get down to my old 9½ to 10 stone and wear size 12 jeans again, but I know the result of such drastic weight loss in someone my age – seventy at my next birthday – would do no favours to my face.

I don't want to insult the former chancellor of the exchequer Nigel Lawson, who lost a huge amount of weight through dieting and phenomenal self-control, but I have found myself saying, 'I don't want to look like Nigel Lawson.' His face rather crumpled with extreme weight loss and he seemed to age ten years in a very short space of time.

It was Dame Barbara Cartland who told me many years ago, when she was ninety years old, 'After forty a woman has to choose between her face and her figure. My advice is to keep a plump pretty face and stay sitting down.' The former model and Oscar-nominated actor Candice Bergen gave similar advice in her memoir, *A Fine Romance*. At the age of sixty-eight, she merrily admitted that over the past sixteen years she had put on nearly 2 stone, loved her food and couldn't understand why her contemporaries either starved or vomited to remain stick-thin.

Of course, there's a world of difference between obesity and a bit of plumptitude. I'm now completely happy to be a bit buxom and have my slightly round, chubby, cheery face, which has not yet collapsed into miserable, thin, pinched wrinkles. I hope to stay this way for the rest of my life, which I'm sure will be longer than it would have been without the surgery.

I've stopped serving my food on large plates. My small portions looked ridiculous on a full-size dinner plate. I haven't completely given up drinking alcohol and still enjoy the occasional glass of good red wine or a vodka and Fever-Tree slimline tonic, but no one is allowed to say or even think 'wine o'clock' in my house. I truly have learned to listen to my appetite and eat only when I'm hungry and stop when I'm full.

I enjoy my food and I know, from what some less fortunate fellow gastric surgery patients have told me, that I'm lucky that my change in eating patterns has not made me find less pleasure in it. I still love dinner with the family or out with a friend, and I can't think of any food that my stomach would reject. Some patients say they can no longer eat bread because it makes them feel sick. I can, but never more than half a slice at a sitting and always brown, or that delicious Irish soda bread. It's quality and portion size that count for me.

I've learned not to feel guilty about wasting food and have managed to shake off what would have been my mother's appalled comments if I hadn't cleaned my plate. If there's too much on it for me to cope with, I give it to my husband to finish, throw it away or, if we're in a restaurant, I ask for a doggy bag. Butch, Frieda and Madge are thrilled that I often come home with a little treat for them.

There's only one thing that really annoys me since I became so much slimmer. People I haven't seen for a while look at me as if they barely recognize me. 'Gosh,' they say, 'you look wonderful. Have you lost weight?' To which I long to reply, 'Yes, are you saying that I looked revolting before?' I don't say it, ever; I simply smile, gratefully and apparently flattered. I nod in agreement, but I do think people should be more aware of how they're playing into that damaging stigma when they imply a fat woman is by definition ugly. She's not.

Conclusion

Do I have any regrets about being seen as someone who 'took the easy way out' to lose weight? Not for one second have I had any doubts that I did exactly the right thing for me. Nor will I have anyone suggest to my face that surgery is an easy cop-out of the arduous work of losing it the conventional way by dieting. It's very frightening to place yourself in the hands of a man or woman with a scalpel and trust them to get it right. It's terrifying, no matter how well you've got to know and like them. It's scary to be in hospital and have part of your body changed for ever without any real certainty that the result will be what you're hoping for. In my case, I was extremely lucky. I got the right surgeon, the right support and the result I had longed for, but it was hard.

Nor was it easy to learn to trust the newly reduced stomach, and learn what it was able to cope with and what it really was not able to accept. It has meant sticking as strictly as possible to new dietary rules, trying out the occasional foray into a steak, which always has to be small and requires a great deal of chewing, and hoping I won't regurgitate it or even be sick. I learned to resist the rich puddings friends encouraged me to consume, allowing myself only a very occasional tasty 'treat', and generally feeling an immense sense of relief that I was not going to starve, even as the pounds fell away. It did, though, begin to be a pleasure to go out for dinner with my naturally slender friends whose portions had always been much tinier than mine and see them look on in amazement as I consumed far less than they did! Those hunger hormones are certainly at bay.

I have to say, though, that the much harder way of trying to lose weight was all those ghastly diets during which I could never truly relax and enjoy all the pleasures that food brings, and which I'd been taught to love and appreciate from when I was tiny. I do regret never having found a way, years ago, of meeting informed experts who would really be able to teach me about the body's biology and the scientific discoveries that have made us understand why we get fat, why dieting can make us obese and ill, and what harm we do to ourselves by eating what we think will be healthy, but ain't necessarily so.

I relied so often on what turned out to be snake-oil salesmen, publishing their diet books and making vast amounts of money, but not really comprehending the way the body responds to certain foods and what happens when you follow a fad diet, reach your goal and then have to give up because your body seems to turn on you and make you more hungry than you ever imagined possible.

And we do give up, as I've said, unless we have a cast-iron will and the time and energy to drag ourselves out, day after day, to the pool, the gym or the running track. For so many of us, that kind of self-denial and determination is impossible to achieve and sustain, especially if, at the same time as trying to restrict our own intake of food and train as heartily as Mo Farah, we are working hard to earn the money to put food on the table for our families and cooking it the rest of the time to give them wonderful nutrition and pleasure.

Food is one of the greatest joys in life and it's something we experience early on. It's not only the look of love on the faces of our parents that makes us realize what delight they find in putting something delicious in front of us. The vital role food plays in all our lives is evident everywhere and all the time from the moment we are born. The first time we are put to the breast or the bottle gives us that comforting experience of skin-to-skin contact with someone who loves us enough to hold us close and provide sustenance. Grandmas and grand-pas bring chocolate and sweets to give us enjoyment, and even the early literature we read often has food at its centre.

For the very small there are picture books such as *The Very Hungry Caterpillar* by Eric Carle. In one week he eats an enor-mous amount of stuff – he goes through an apple, two pears, three plums, four strawberries, five oranges, a piece of choc-olate cake, an ice-cream cone, a pickle, a slice of Swiss cheese, a slice of salami, a lollipop, a piece of cherry pie, a sausage, a cupcake and a slice of watermelon. He grows and grows and becomes a little plump, forms a chrysalis, sleeps for a fortnight and emerges as a large, beautiful butterfly.

Similarly, in Judith Kerr's *The Tiger Who Came to Tea*, the tiger turns up at Sophie's home at teatime. He drinks all the tea, eats every scrap of food he can find in the house and even drains every drop of water from the taps. It's often been said that Kerr wrote the book as an echo of the time she spent in Berlin as a small child, when her father was on a Nazi death list, before they escaped to London. Speculation has suggested that she invented the tiger because she understood that people could turn up at your house and take away everything you cared about.

'Not a bit of it,' she told me. The idea came after a trip to see the tigers at the zoo and she thought it would amuse her daughter to think of a friendly, fun tiger turning up at the house, scoffing everything, leaving peacefully and then, when Daddy came home and there was nothing to eat, the family would go out to a restaurant for sausages, chips and ice cream. The tiger's greed led to a great treat for the family. Then, the following day, Sophie and her mother go shopping and bring back a big tin of tiger food, but the tiger doesn't return.

It seems to me these books are so universally popular and beloved because they take our children's first and fundamental source of sensual pleasure – delicious food – and say, it's OK, it's there to be enjoyed. Most children love to be given new things to eat. The food sits on the plate, is touched and played with, tasted, and either rejected because the flavour doesn't suit or consumed hungrily, rolled around the tongue as the taste buds discover the delightful sensations that eating lovely things can switch on.

For older children there's a literary source that emphasizes how awful it is to have no parents and always to be hungry. Charles Dickens' Oliver Twist is an orphan, raised until the age of nine under the terms of the Poor Law in a baby farm and then sent to the workhouse where the children are starving. Oliver draws lots with the other boys to decide who will ask for another bowl of gruel. He gets the short straw, has to do the unenviable job, and speaks some of the most famous words in the English language to Mr Bumble: 'Please, sir, I want some more.' Bad food and lack of good nourishment means childhood cruelty and potential disaster. It's a powerful lesson that Dickens introduces to his readers, both young and old.

So, literature frequently puts the love of food at the centre of our cultural lives when we are young. Then, look what happens when we are grown. On television we see Paul Hollywood and Prue Leith give a group of amateur bakers seemingly impossible tasks to complete on *The Great British Bake Off*. The contestants have to demonstrate their technical skills and then turn cakes, buns, biscuits and bread into exotic works of art. It's a carb (and sugar) fest at the end of each programme as Prue and Paul tuck into endless examples of sweet and starchy stuff, generally with relish. And on it goes. A week rarely passes without *Masterchef*, *Celebrity Masterchef*, *The Hairy Bikers*, *Saturday Kitchen* and *Nadiya's Summer Feasts* – I recently had a difficult time resisting going out to buy golden syrup to try to emulate her recipe for baklava, once my favourite sweet, traditionally a combination of filo pastry, nuts and honey. It would have been interesting to try her golden-syrup version, but *no*!

Then there are the chefs Nigel Slater, Mary Berry, Jamie Oliver, Gordon Ramsay and Tom Kerridge, frequently on TV and often invited to *Woman's Hour* to cook a perfect dish. Nigel's apple pie is already on record as being the best ever, Mary's lemon meringue pie is truly to die for, and Jamie managed to get away with calling me 'darlin', perhaps because he cooked the most wonderful collection of Italian delights. It's a constant temptation to try to copy these great cooks and chefs, and a never-ending reminder of how central the consumption of fancy food has become, both at home and in restaurants.

I remember the days when the average family couldn't afford to go out for a blow-out and, even if they could, the fare tended to be somewhat limited. Maybe there'd be a Brown Windsor soup, a roast, two veg and some gravy, and an apple pie on offer. There'd be none of the international exotica to which we now have such easy access, whether it be sitting down in a restaurant or having a takeaway delivered to the door. For that, there is barely any exercise involved at all – you hardly have to get up from the sofa.

There's a bizarre contradiction going on at the moment. On the one hand, food is fashionable. It's not only the constant barrage of people on television continually concocting delicious things to eat, Jay Rayner and his guests on *The Kitchen Cabinet* also do it on the radio. There's Instagram and Twitter, those social-media show-off centres, where a constant stream of photos are posted by anyone and everyone – some famous, most not – displaying what goodies they've put on their plate that day.

At the same time as Instagram and the popular press advertise the fabulous food that can be made at home, they're also all full of the current weight-loss heroes, whether its Tom Watson, Tom Kerridge, Gordon Ramsay, Kim Kardashian, Susanna Reid, Adele, Oprah Winfrey (again) or the women who got their slender bodies back mere days after having a baby. It's enough to make us all feel hopelessly inadequate if we are not cordon-bleu cooks alongside what's considered to be the perfect size and shape.

Most disturbing, together with the trend for pushing the somewhat pornographic aspects of food, is the never-ending promotion of fear of fatness and ill health. In the *Daily Mail*, for example, you'll find a banner headline that reads 'Free magazine: What to eat to beat diabetes – with NHS diabetes expert', followed on page one by 'Failure of food firms to slash sugar "woeful"'.

This particular report, published by Public Health England in May 2018, praised the efforts of the drinks industry to reduce sugar content, but said that in some foods, including biscuits and chocolate, levels had gone up and it was Professor Susan Jebb, the government's former 'obesity tsar', who had described the industry's efforts as 'woeful'. She also said, 'We need a new approach if we are serious about reducing sugar and calories from confectionery. This can't be left to businesses. We need new policies to persuade people to eat less or to stop encouraging them to eat more.' She stressed that two-thirds of adults in Britain and a third of children are overweight.

When Professor Dame Sally Davies, the outgoing chief medical officer for England, published her final report in 2019, she rather underlined her nickname, 'the nanny-in-chief', when she concentrated on the obesity crisis and advocated a ban on eating on public transport, a ban on promoting and advertising junk food, and raising VAT on foods that are high in salt, sugar or fat. Her proposal would have prevented a deal that had been struck that same week between the England and Wales Cricket Board and KP Snacks.

Her concern, she said, was for children, and she was alarmed that England was nowhere near the government's goal of halving obesity rates by 2030. She was deeply worried that 10 in every 30 primary-school children are now overweight or obese. She was convinced the public would be behind her proposals because there is support for the government to protect children.

I can't deny that she's on the right lines, as we've seen how children – particularly in poorer areas – are bombarded with adverts and restaurants promoting junk food. Maybe banning eating and drinking on public transport was a little over the top. Even with my reduced appetite, I'd find a long train journey a trial without some access to something to eat!

There was more in the same edition of the *Daily Mail* that carried the articles on diabetes and sugar. Later in the paper, there was a feature that began, 'Shockingly, 3.4 million Britons have type 2 diabetes.' The wife of the chef Giancarlo Caldesi declared, 'Honey, I shrunk my husband (and you can too!),' and the doctor who helped her with his diet, David Unwin, gave a list of what can and can't be included in a low-carb diet.

1. Reduce or eliminate your intake of sugar and high-carb foods, including breakfast cereals, bread, pasta, white potatoes, rice, couscous, crackers, oats, oat cakes, rice cakes, cakes, biscuits, sweets, milk chocolate, fruit juice, fizzy drinks and cordials.
2. At every meal load up with non-starchy and salad vegetables such as kale, lettuce, broccoli, mushrooms or peppers.
3. Eat good fats, including oily fish, olive oil, coconut oil, avocado and animal fats. Add nuts and cheese in moderation – although nutritious, they are high in calories.
4. Choose fruit naturally low in sugar – including berries, apples and pears – over high-sugar tropical fruits such as bananas, mango and pineapple.
5. Eat some form of protein at every meal.
6. Stop snacking. Fasting between meals and overnight helps improve your body's response to insulin.
7. Drink 2 litres of water a day to keep your body well-hydrated.
   NOTE: Always consult your GP before starting a new diet plan, particularly if taking any medication.

I felt like screaming, '*We know!*' I do not underestimate the extent of obesity and type 2 diabetes, the pressure it places on the NHS and the need for us all to be aware of the potential danger it causes us. *But*. . . I think many of those lucky people among us who are naturally thin, and in that I include a lot of GPs, have no idea of the painful effort involved in self-denial when so much wonderful food is consistently paraded in front of us. I think too that a lot of members of the medical profession are not as aware as they should be of the genetic and metabolic science I've discussed in this book. And if they're not aware, how can we be aware?

Curiously, only two days after the double-page spread on how to diet to beat diabetes, and in the same newspaper's Sunday edition, came a huge article headlined, 'Why the woman who told us all to quit sugar now eats cake and chocolate.'

The *Mail* interview was carried out by Eve Simmons, one of the authors of *Eat It Anyway: Fight the Food Fads, Beat Anxiety and Eat in Peace*. Simmons, who's suffered from eating disorders in the past, points to her awareness of the links between restrictive eating and serious mental illness. She quotes the eating-disorder psychiatrist Dr Mark Berelowitz, who revealed in 2016 that what he considered a shocking 80–90 per cent of the patients attending his North London clinic were avid followers of bloggers and social-media stars who advised avoiding entire food groups, including sugar.

Just as Professor Rubino was concerned by the lack of scientific evidence that sugar is the main dietary enemy, Eve Simmons also worries about the danger of excluding any food group from one's diet and breaks down some of the myths surrounding sugar. 'Clearly,' she writes, 'a diet heavy in sugary doughnuts and fizzy drinks won't do wonders for our health. But studies show that, provided we don't eat bucket loads of it, sugar is perfectly fine in the diet.'

There is no evidence that sugar alone causes obesity. There is evidence that high-sugar diets are also typically high in fats, salt and numerous sources of calories, so it's impossible to pinpoint which of them causes weight gain. It's generally accepted that it's simply too much of everything that causes us to become obese.

Similarly, even though type 2 diabetes leads to raised blood sugar levels, there is no evidence it happens simply because sugar is eaten. It's being overweight or obese that is the primary factor in developing the disease, regardless of what we have eaten. As we've seen from the most recent research into metabolic science, it's excess fat in the liver that appears to mess up the body's endocrine system. It's not just sugar but, I repeat, too much of everything that creates the problems.

It is a fact that we can become addicted to the pleasure of food – it's what we call comfort eating. It cheers us when we're down. It's exactly the same psychological impulse that might drive us to crave alcohol, heroin, nicotine or cannabis to brighten our day or relax us. But we don't actually need any of those drugs. We can, perhaps with some psychological assistance or the support of an organization such as Alcoholics Anonymous, give them up completely without harming ourselves physically in any way. Food is a much bigger problem for us to regulate because without it, we die.

Nevertheless, the constant criticism of fat people, which creates the debilitating stigma, continues apace. In early September 2019, the American comedian and political commentator Bill Maher told the audience of his TV show *Real Time* that 'fat shaming doesn't need to end. It needs to make a comeback.' He added: 'Shame is the first step in reform.'

Piers Morgan, presenting *Good Morning Britain*, echoed Maher's view and said he had 'rightly outlined a problem. What has Bill Maher said that was wrong? We've become a society now where we don't just tolerate morbid obesity, we celebrate it. Stop celebrating being massively overweight. I don't know how you get people to lose weight unless you say, "Come on. Enough." I think the best way to lose weight is when someone goes, "Blimey, you've put on a bit, son." So you feel a bit insecure and then you go off and reduce one Big Mac a day to half a Big Mac and so you go on.'

James Corden, best known for *Gavin and Stacey* and now host of *The Late Late Show* in the US, hit back at Maher and Morgan on his own talk show, with a background overlay to the side of him that read 'Fat Shaming'. On Twitter he wrote, 'If making fun of fat people made them lose weight, there'd be no fat kids in school.' On his programme he said that fat shaming never went anywhere. 'I mean, ask literally any fat person. We are reminded of it all the time. There is a common and insulting misconception that fat people are stupid and lazy. It is proven that fat shaming only does one thing – it makes people feel ashamed. And shame leads to depression, anxiety and self-destructive behaviour. Self-destructive behaviour like overeating.'

I am somewhat conflicted on this question because, had it not been for Charlie's anxiety that I might become like the woman in the park, disabled by being so overweight, I might never have summoned up the courage to seek a solution to my problem. His intention was not cruel fat shaming, but a son's genuine concern for his mother's health and wellbeing, and he did prompt me to act. At the same time, though, I know from long and bitter experience that being called a 'fat cow' by strangers in the street never made me anything other than miserable and upset and motivated to run to the next bite of comfort food. It's difficult.

So how would I have proceeded throughout my life if I'd known in the early days what I know now? I would have ignored my mother's sniffy comments about how it was such a pity that I'd inherited my father's heavy bone structure rather than her fine one, and I would have learned to live in my own body without feeling I had to criticize my appearance constantly. I would also have accepted that I didn't have to be super-slim to be healthy.

Most importantly, I would have said 'no' to her on all those days when I was forced to eat more than I wanted. As a child and a teenager, I did naturally what Susie Orbach has always advised. I listened to my appetite and, when it told me to stop, I would have stopped, had my mother and grandmother not insisted that enormous portions of their lovely food were essential and nothing should be wasted.

That would be my advice to parents. Never criticize your child's size, never force food upon them that they really don't want because they're not hungry (maybe a little insistence on vegetables might be permissible) and feed them a range of foods, excluding nothing, in sensibly small portions. Try not to portray sweets and chocolates as 'treats', but just something that you can eat occasionally. It's also essential that parents never pass their own anxieties about their weight and habits of constant dieting on to their children. My mother dieted all the time and when she wasn't encouraging me to stuff myself, she was cutting out anything from our diet that might make either of us fat. It led to an unhealthy relationship with food, which only my surgery has managed to regulate. We must all feel entitled to eat and feel no fear of anything, accepting that eating should be a pleasure and never a guilty one.

I remember another piece of advice from Susie Orbach that has stayed with me throughout most of my adult life: 'Beauty comes in many sizes.' I'm reminded of it often when I walk my little dogs in the park. They are beautiful small Chihuahuas. Butch, the oldest and only male, is quite big – about the size of a Jack Russell. Frieda is considerably smaller and Madge, the youngest, is smaller still – diminutive, in fact. People often stop us to say, 'Aah! They're so cute. What breeds are they?' I explain they're all Chihuahuas. 'But why is the white one so much bigger than the others,' they ask, 'if they're all the same breed?' I'm afraid I find myself saying, 'Well, we're the same breed. Human beings. Why do you suppose I'm so much bigger (or, very occasionally, smaller) than you?'

I don't go on about genes and hormones and metabolism, about the science and psychology of it all. I just say, 'That's the way it is and it's absolutely fine.'

Bibliography

Crockett, R. A., King, S. E., Marteau, T. M., Prevost, A. T., Bignardi, G., Roberts, N. W., and Jebb, S. A. (2018), 'Nutritional labelling for healthier food or non-alcoholic drink purchasing and consumption', *The Cochrane Database of Systematic Reviews*, 2 (2).

Hagan, S. (2019), *Happy Fat: Taking Up Space in a World That Wants to Shrink You* (London: 4th Estate).

Ingalls, A. M., Dickie, M. M., and Snell, G. D. (1950), 'Obese, a new mutation in the house mouse', *Journal of Heredity*, 41 (12), 317–18.

Mann, T. (2017), *Secrets from the Eating Lab: The Science of Weight Loss, the Myth of Willpower and Why You Should Never Diet Again* (London: Harper Wave).

Orbach, S. (2006), *Fat Is a Feminist Issue* (London: Arrow).

Pattison, J. (2017), *The Healthy Gut Handbook* (London: Seven Dials).

Schwimmer, J. B., Burwinkle, T. M., and Varni, J. W. (2003), 'Health-related quality of life of severely obese children and adolescents', *Journal of the American Medical Association*, 289 (14), 1813–19.

Simmons, E., and Dennison, L. (2019), *Eat It Anyway: Fight the Food Fads, Beat Anxiety and Eat in Peace* (London: Mitchell Beazley).

Spector, T. (2015), *The Diet Myth: The Real Science Behind What We Eat* (London: Weidenfeld & Nicolson).

Warner, A. (2019), *The Truth About Fat* (London: Oneworld).

Watson, H. J., Yilmaz, Z., Thornton, L. M. *et al.* (2019), 'Genome-wide association study identifies eight risk loci and implicates metabo-psychiatric origins for anorexia nervosa', *Nature Genetics*, 51, 1207–14.

Yeo, G. (2018), *Gene Eating* (London: Orion Spring).

Acknowledgements

I could not have written this book without the help of fellow sufferers from obesity who shared their struggles with me frankly and often painfully. Emma Burnell made the journey across London to join me for coffee, and Nigel Payne and Tom Kerridge gave me lots of time on the phone. Some asked me not to use their real names, which I have respected. I am grateful to them all.

For assistance in understanding the science of obesity and weight loss I must first thank Dr Giles Yeo. We have never met, but I have drawn information from his book *Gene Eating* quite ruthlessly. It's a book I've reread frequently in my attempts to understand the way my own body works and why it has caused me so much grief.

Professors David Cummings and Rebecca Puhl gave their time freely in transatlantic phone calls, and Rebecca sent a mass of her research papers on the impact of stigma for me to read. Professor Roy Taylor was not so far away. Phone calls to him only stretched as far as Newcastle.

I must mention Dr Billy White here, as he was the person who first led me to research the science of obesity, but my most heartfelt thanks go to Professor Francesco Rubino, who has always been available on the phone and face to face to give me information, understanding and support.

Thanks go to my professional support network – my lovely literary agent Barbara Levy, my attentive and, at times, rightly demanding editor Andrea Henry, and my equally fastidious and excellent copy editor Rebecca Wright.

Last but not least, my family: David, Ed and Charlie, who loved and supported me thin or fat.

About the Author

Jenni Murray is a journalist and broadcaster who presented BBC Radio 4's *Woman's Hour* from 1987 to 2020. She is the author of several books and writes a weekly column in the *Daily Mail*. She lives in north London and the New Forest.